O D L
OXFORD DIABETES LIBRARY

Type 1 Diabetes

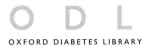

O D L
OXFORD DIABETES LIBRARY

Type 1 Diabetes

David Levy

Consultant Physician, Gillian Hanson Centre
for Diabetes and Endocrinology, Whipps Cross
University Hospital, London, UK
Hon Senior Lecturer, Queen Mary University
of London

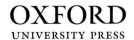

OXFORD
UNIVERSITY PRESS

OXFORD
UNIVERSITY PRESS

Great Clarendon Street, Oxford OX2 6DP

Oxford University Press is a department of the University of Oxford.
It furthers the University's objective of excellence in research, scholarship,
and education by publishing worldwide in

Oxford New York

Auckland Cape Town Dar es Salaam Hong Kong Karachi
Kuala Lumpur Madrid Melbourne Mexico City Nairobi
New Delhi Shanghai Taipei Toronto

With offices in

Argentina Austria Brazil Chile Czech Republic France Greece
Guatemala Hungary Italy Japan Poland Portugal Singapore
South Korea Switzerland Thailand Turkey Ukraine Vietnam

Oxford is a registered trade mark of Oxford University Press
in the UK and in certain other countries

Published in the United States
by Oxford University Press Inc., New York

British Library Cataloguing in Publication Data

Data available

Library of Congress Cataloging in Publication Data

Data available

Typeset by Newgen Imaging Systems (P) Ltd., Chennai, India
Printed in Great Britain
on acid-free paper by
Ashford Colour Press Ltd., Gosport, Hampshire

ISBN 978–0–19–955321–1

10 9 8 7 6 5 4 3 2 1

Whilst every effort has been made to ensure that the contents of this book are as
complete, accurate, and up-to-date as possible at the date of writing. Oxford
University Press is not able to give any guarantee or assurance that such is the case.
Readers are urged to take appropriately qualified medical advice in all cases. The
information in this book is intended to be useful to the general reader, but should
not be used as a means of self-diagnosis or for the prescription of medication.

Contents

Preface

Writing a short, contemporary, practical book on Type 1 diabetes is a challenge. Secondary care teams do not need me to tell them how important glycaemic control is. However, the evidence for the primacy of glycaemia is overwhelming, and much of this book concentrates on why and how we must do better. No book, however large, could encompass all the individual strategies we use every day. Conversely, the guidelines-heavy approach now gloomily familiar in Type 2 diabetes practice is inappropriate, because Type 1 diabetes is guidelines-lite (at least at present), largely because it is relatively light on evidence. There was no point including molecular mechanisms in a practical pocket book, even if I knew anything about them. (One reviewer of the book's outline questioned whether books had any relevance at all in an electronic age to rapidly-developing subjects such as diabetes, a wider issue I do not have space to tackle here—perhaps that was the point he was making. Actually, I do not believe that clinically important aspects of Type 1 diabetes arrive quite so frequently, and even if they did the necessary delay and consideration involved in a printed summary has real benefits in a world where articles e-pubbed months before print frequently overwhelm rather than inform or guide.) Finally, heavy pharmacology was not needed. Those of us who enjoy the challenges of Type 1 diabetes also appreciate its therapeutic parsimony: insulin, and in many, not much besides (though the potential for new technology, especially pumps and continuous glucose monitors, is remarkable).

Recognizing these limits, which should have resulted in a very short book indeed, I have highlighted some themes that I hope will stimulate teams managing Type 1 diabetes. For example, while clinically significant microvascular complications may be declining, macrovascular complications are emerging in people with long-standing diabetes who thankfully have escaped the ravages of nephropathy. The management of this important group is not known—but aware and vigilant we must be. Other important areas are diabetes in adolescence, the important period of emerging adulthood, psychological problems, especially in younger people, and at the other end of life, the poorly covered problems of the elderly with Type 1 diabetes. Apart from the last, the literature in these areas is impressive, even if translation into practice has been weak, and I have tried to summarize knowledge using up to date sources.

No apology is needed for continual reference to the Diabetes Control and Complications Trial (DCCT) and its follow-up, Epidemiology of Diabetes Interventions and Complications (EDIC). Revelatory publications still pour from this study, in my view the greatest clinical trial in medicine, its status immeasurably enhanced by the exemplary democracy of the DCCT Research Group in opening up the study databanks to independent researchers worldwide.

Trainees interested in the acute problems of Type 1 diabetes might be attracted by the chapters on long-term complications. Awareness of Type 1 diabetes in primary care is important, and advanced practitioners may find something of interest here. Finally, a concise, selective approach may appeal to medical students, though we were all agreed that T-cell immunology should not be here. I have included PubMed PMID numbers for journal references, and entered as their unique seven- or eight-digit number into the search window of pubmed.gov should give instant access to abstracts, especially useful for guidelines, consensus statements, and DDCT/EDIC Research Group publications, which often have inconsistent reference styles.

I was rash enough to write all the chapters, and am responsible for their content, but they have been extensively revised after review by brave experts who will have gnashed their teeth seeing their life's work condensed into a few, albeit after their efforts I hope crystalline, sentences. I am particularly grateful to my good friend Dr. Tore Julsrud Berg (Aker University Hospital, Oslo) for his detailed review of the whole manuscript, but especially Chapters 4 and 5 which have benefited from his extraordinary experience. Dr. Henrik Ullits Andersen (Steno Diabetes Centre, Gentofte) was another kindly reviewer. Laura Liew, with her usual stunning efficiency, virtually kept me to deadlines, took photographs, and helped with case histories, tables, and line diagrams. The sections on CSII were bracingly enhanced by Laila King (London Medical, Marylebone). Nic Wilson and Jenny Wright of OUP cornered me once in my office and demanded, most charmingly, that I hand over the manuscript. They have been very supportive, and I thank Nic, Peter Stevenson and the OUP delegates for embarking on this project with a jobbing diabetologist.

David Levy
July 2010

Symbols and abbreviations

↓	decreased
↑	increased
ABPM	ambulatory BP monitoring
AcAc	acetoacetate
ACEi	angiotensin converting enzyme inhibitor
ACR	albumin:creatinine ratio
ACS	acute coronary syndrome
ADA	American Diabetes Association
AER	albumin excretion rate
AGEs	advanced glycation end products
AITD	autoimmune thyroid disease
APECED	autoimmune polyendocrinopathy, candidiasis, ectodermal dysplasia
APS	autoimmune polyglandular syndromes
BMI	body mass index
BP	blood pressure
CAC	coronary artery calcification
CAD	coronary artery disease
CAPD	continuous ambulatory peritoneal dialysis
CETP	cholesteryl ester transfer protein
CGM	continuous glucose monitoring
CIMT	carotid intima–media thickness
CKD	chronic kidney disease
CNS	central nervous system
CRP	C-reactive protein
CSF	cerebrospinal fluid
CSII	continuous subcutaneous insulin infusion
CT	computed tomography
CTS	carpal tunnel syndrome
DASH	Dietary Approaches to Stop Hypertension
DCCT	Diabetes Control and Complications Trial

DIRECT	DIabetic Retinopathy Candesartan Trials
DKA	diabetic ketoacidosis
eAG	estimated average glucose
ECG	electrocardiogram
EDIC	Epidemiology of Diabetes Interventions and Complications
ENDIT	European Nicotinamide Diabetes Intervention Trial
ESRD	end-stage renal disease
GADA	glutamic acid decarboxylase antibodies
GFR	glomerular filteration rate
eGFR	estimated glomerular filteration rate
GH	growth hormone
GIK	glucose–insulin–potassium
HAAF	hypoglycaemia-associated autonomic failure
HDL	high-density lipoprotein
HLA	human leukocyte antigen
HOMA-IR	homeostasis model assessment of insulin resistance
IAA	insulin autoantibodies
ICA	islet-cell antibodies
IDDM	insulin-dependent diabetes mellitus
IGF-I	insulin-like growth factor I
IL	interleukin
IRMA	intraretinal microvascular abnormalities
LADA	latent autoimmune diabetes of adults
LCAT	lecithin cholesterol acyl transferase
LDL	low-density lipoprotein
LGV	large goods vehicles
MDI	multiple daily injections
MDNS	Michigan Diabetic Neuropathy Score
MNSI	Michigan Neuropathy Screening Instrument
MPI	myocardial perfusion imaging
MRI	magnetic resonance imaging
MRSA	methicillin-resistant *Staphylococcus aureus*
NCEP-ATP	National Cholesterol Education Program, Adult Treatment Panel

NF	nuclear factor
NPDR	non-proliferative diabetic retinopathy
NPH	neutral protamine Hagedorn
OCT	optical coherence tomography
β-OHB	β-hydroxybutyrate
PA	pernicious anaemia
PAK	pancreas-after-kidney
PCOS	polycystic ovarian syndrome
PCV	passenger-carrying vehicles
PDR	proliferative diabetic retinopathy
PVD	peripheral vascular disease
PZI	protamine zinc insulin
QoL	quality of life
RCT	randomized controlled trial
ROS	reactive oxygen species
SPK	simultaneous pancreas kidney
SMBG	self-monitoring of blood glucose
STEMI	ST segment elevation myocardial infarction
TB	tuberculosis
TNF	tissue necrosis factor
UVB	ultraviolet B
VEGF	vascular endothelial growth factor

Chapter 1

Classification and aetiology

Key points

- Type 1 diabetes is a common complex autoimmune condition especially prevalent in Caucasian white northern and southern populations.
- Incidence is increasing rapidly, especially in the under 5 age group; cases are likely to double in northern countries between 2005 and 2020.
- High-risk human leucocyte antigen haplotypes are carried by more than 90% of Type 1 patients; protective haplotypes also exist.
- Latent autoimmune diabetes in adults (LADA) is frequent in older people with phenotypic features of Type 2 diabetes. It is an important diagnosis to make whenever possible at onset to raise awareness of the requirement for insulin treatment.
- Tests for islet antibodies (glutamic acid decarboxylase, islet cell, and IA-2) can be valuable in the diagnosis of LADA, and are used to rapidly screen large high-risk populations.
- Up to now, primary and secondary intervention trials have been mostly unsuccessful, but tertiary intervention in the period immediately following clinical diagnosis shows much more promise, and an international programme (www.diabetestrialnet.org) of clinical trials in newly-diagnosed patients (and studies of prevention in close relatives) is exploring new interventional agents.

1

1.1 Historical

Clinical recognition of diabetes long preceded the realization that the pancreas was frequently damaged in patients with the condition. This occurred in the middle of the 19th century. Claude Bernard (1813–1878) discovered experimentally that both the liver and the brain were involved in glucose metabolism. Paul Langerhans (1847–1888) in 1869, and Gustave-Eduard Laguesse in 1893, hinted, through their recognition of the pancreatic islets of Langerhans (Laguesse named them) at a dual function of the pancreas, now known to be endocrine and exocrine, and this was confirmed in 1889 when Minkowski and von Mering, and then definitively Hédon, in 1893, discovered that pancreatectomized dogs developed diabetes after rigorously excluding pancreatic exocrine secretion. Even in 1922, when Banting, Best, Collip, and Macleod first used insulin therapeutically, the confusion between the two functions of the pancreas initially blurred their experimental design. In 1935, Dorothy Hodgkin (1910–1994) obtained the first X-ray crystallography pictures of insulin, but the full crystalline structure was not revealed for another 34 yrs. In 1955, Frederick Sanger (b. 1918) sequenced its amino acids. Thereafter technological discoveries came rapidly: radioimmunoassay was first used to measure serum insulin in 1958, the insulin receptor was characterized in the early 1970s, and the insulin gene sequence in 1980. However, the autoimmune nature of Type 1 diabetes was not established until the work of Doniach and Bottazzo in 1979.

The terrible and lingering death suffered by countless young people until the early 1920s at the hands of well-meaning physicians with only the most rudimentary notions of intermediary metabolism, and the remarkable results of insulin treatment, even with the crude preparations available in the early days, is the greatest example of 20th-century clinical medical science. The detailed story, related in Michael Bliss's *The Discovery of Insulin* (Bliss 2007) should be read by everyone involved in the care of people with diabetes.

1.2 Nomenclature

The designation Type 1 diabetes is relatively recent (1998). It was previously defined in terms of treatment and its mandatory nature—insulin-dependent diabetes—and previously, perhaps more obviously, by its age of onset, characteristically in the young—hence juvenile-onset diabetes. The cumbersome term Type 1 (insulin-dependent) diabetes was used in the 1990s; the euphonious acronym insulin-dependent diabetes mellitus (IDDM) should no longer be used. Simple tests of autoimmunity in widespread use have expanded the spectrum of Type 1 diabetes, but the autoimmune process still cannot be identified in a small group of patients; non-autoimmune Type 1 diabetes has been termed Type 1B, while the overwhelmingly more common form should technically be termed Type 1A diabetes. Further discussion of the clinical presentation of these sub-types can be found in Chapter 2.

1.3 Epidemiology

1.3.1 Age and gender

As well as Type 1 diabetes, other unrelated immune diseases, including multiple sclerosis, Crohn's disease, and asthma, have substantially increased over the past three decades, in striking contrast to the continued fall in infectious diseases (e.g. measles, mumps, tuberculosis (TB), rheumatic fever, and hepatitis A) over the same period. There is some epidemiological and much experimental evidence to support a causal link between the two trends—the 'hygiene hypothesis'.

Its peak incidence is between 10 and 15 yrs, somewhat earlier in girls than boys. Studies consistently show a more rapid rise in incidence in the under 5s compared with older children up to 16. Recent data from Finland, which has an exceptionally high level of Type 1 diabetes, documents a doubling in the rate of childhood diabetes between 1980 and 2005, and projects a further doubling between 2005 and 2020 (Harjutsalo *et al.* 2008). There is no evidence that this increased rate in young people is being balanced by a lower rate in older groups (the so-called spring harvest). The 'accelerator hypothesis' has been proposed to explain the increased incidence in young children (and also a unifying hypothesis for both Type 1 and Type 2 diabetes); it proposes that rapidly increasing levels of obesity in western populations lead to earlier exposure of borderline insulin deficiency in the overweight and insulin resistant—and therefore earlier presentation in the obese child (Wilkin 2008). Good evidence for this in the UK has recently been challenged by contradictory findings in Australia.

From adolescence onwards, the incidence gradually decreases up to age 30, though there is a small peak around age 40. However, this long 'tail' contains the majority of patients diagnosed with Type 1 diabetes. Male preponderance emerges from age 15, and is at its most marked in the 25 to 29 age group. In most countries the male:female ratio in this age group is >1.5, unique and unexplained for an autoimmune disease, where there is usually a substantial female excess.

1.3.2 Geographical

Incidence of Type 1 diabetes increases strongly with increasing latitude; Finland has the highest incidence in the world (though the human leucocyte antigen (HLA)-similar population of Sardinia has a similar incidence), but even within a relatively small country such as the UK, there is still a pronounced north–south gradient—for example, the incidence in Scotland is higher than in England. Both genetic and environmental factors might account for such differences. The incidence also falls dramatically moving eastwards, and the prevalence rates in Asia are very low, for example 0.1 to 0.3/100,000 in China. Between Finland and China, there is a 350-fold difference in incidence in children; across Europe, a tenfold difference. In the nothern hemisphere there is a consistently higher incidence during the winter and spring months.

Data on migrating populations and the risks of developing Type 1 diabetes in their countries of origin and destination implicates environmental factors (see below) to different degrees in different populations. For example, the incidence of Type 1 diabetes in UK South Asian families who have migrated from Pakistan is now the same as that of non-immigrants, and more than 10 times the incidence in Pakistan. The incidence in Indians in the UK increased nearly fourfold between 1980 and 1990, while Sardinians migrating to Italy maintain the high incidence found in their native island (Leslie *et al.* 2006).

1.4 Causative factors

1.4.1 Genetic factors

Genetic factors are clearly important in determining susceptibility to Type 1 diabetes. For example, while the lifetime risk is 0.4% in those without a family history, this increases to 4–6% in offspring of Type 1 patients (higher risk conferred by fathers compared with mothers in childhood-onset diabetes, but similar risk in adult-onset (15–39 y) diabetes), ~5% in sibs, and up to 50% in identical twins (Harjutsalo *et al.* 2010). All young people with Type 1 diabetes planning a family should be informed of these risks. HLA alleles, on chromosome 6p, are the major determinants of susceptibility to Type 1 diabetes. They encode major histocompatibility class II molecules expressed on the surfaces of antigen-presenting cells, for example macrophages, which in turn present antigens to T cells, the main effectors of the autoimmune process that destroys β-cells.

HLA DR3/DR4 heterozygotes carry the highest risk of developing Type 1 diabetes, and even though this risk is only about 5%, it is more than 15 times the background population risk. More than 90% of Type 1 patients carry one of the following two genotypes: HLA-DR3, DQB1*0201 (also known as DR3-DQ2) or HLA-DR4,DQB1*0302 (DR4-DQ8). Certain DR4 alleles are protective, and decrease the risk, even in the presence of other high-risk alleles.

While useful for population studies, the high rates of these haplotypes in the healthy background population mean that they cannot be used diagnostically; in addition, they decrease in frequency with the age of onset of diabetes. Other genes include those associated with TNF-α and β, IL-10 and IL-6 polymorphisms. Twin studies show a surprisingly low concordance rate, even in young-onset Type 1 diabetes (e.g. 40% to 50%), but this falls to 6% to 25% in older-onset cases, indicating the increasing importance of non-genetic factors.

1.4.2 Environmental factors

The list of postulated environmental factors precipitating or contributing to Type 1 diabetes is long and growing (Box 1.1). While the hygiene hypothesis proposes an increasing risk with decreasing rate of childhood infections, paradoxically, specific enteroviral infections,

> ## Box 1.1 Environmental factors implicated in Type 1 diabetes
>
> - Common to many allergic and autoimmune diseases, including Type 1 diabetes
>   - Increased hygiene/decreased rates of infection
>   - Immunizations
>   - Antibiotics
>   - Increasing prosperity
> - Specific to Type 1 diabetes
>   - Viral infections, especially Coxsackie B4 (associated with seroconversion, and direct effect on β-cell function)
>   - Early exposure to cow's milk
>   - Reduced rates/duration breastfeeding
>   - Vitamin D status and ultraviolet B (UVB) exposure
>   - Nitrite consumption
> - Early exposure to root vegetables or toxic contaminants, for example *Streptomyces* toxins (pleomacrolides)

especially Coxsackie B4, may be responsible for precipitating the onset of Type 1 diabetes in susceptible subjects, via infection of β-cells and inhibition of insulin secretion. In a large Australian population over the past 50 years there has been an increasing penetrance of HLA class II genotypes that previously would have carried a low risk of Type 1 diabetes, though with a continuing high stable level of the usual high-risk genotypes. This striking change reinforces the idea that the environment is playing a more important role in the aetiology of Type 1 diabetes (Fourlanos *et al.* 2008). There is recent interest in the role of vitamin D and ultraviolet B (UVB) radiation. About 25% of the variance in Type 1 diabetes incidence worldwide can be explained by UVB, the main determinant of vitamin D synthesis, and which decreases with increasing geographical latitude. Young adults with Type 1 diabetes have lower serum vitamin D levels than controls, and the weight of evidence is now considered strong enough to support the use of vitamin D supplements during pregnancy and in children after their first year to substantially reduce the incidence of Type 1 diabetes, though the mechanism by which this benefit is mediated is not clear—vitamin D here may be acting as an immunomodulator (Mohr *et al.* 2008).

1.4.3 Autoimmune responses

The autoimmune process leading to islet-cell destruction is associated with a variety of autoantibodies:

- Insulin autoantibodies (IAA)
- Islet-cell antibodies (ICA)
- Insulinoma-associated protein 2 antibodies (IA-2)

- Glutamic acid decarboxylase antibodies (GADA)—GADA is also present in the central nervous system (high-level antibodies associated with the stiff-man/person syndrome) and testes. Note, however, that the background rate of GADA positivity in the background population is ~4%.

It is important to remember that while these autoantibodies are markers of islet-cell destruction there is no evidence that they are of pathogenetic importance either in mediating islet-cell infiltration and inflammation (insulitis) or β-cell destruction. IAA are found more often in childhood-onset diabetes. In late-onset diabetes, GADA are characteristic while IA-2 are rare. ICA are difficult to measure and are not widely used in clinical practice. The presence of combinations of antibodies increases the risk of diabetes in family members who carry them—for example, those positive for all three IAA, GADA, and IA-2 antibodies have a 5-yr risk of ~75%. These combinations are now widely used to screen high-risk patients for potential recruitment into interventional trials (Figure 1.1). However, their presence is not fixed, and varies with age (e.g. GADA were absent in 25% of Belgian Type 1 diabetic patients diagnosed under 40 yrs of age), and their role in differential diagnosis is not clear (see below). Standardizing the methodologies for measuring these antibodies, even GADA, the simplest, still remains troublesome. Even the most dedicated researchers in the field are not convinced that measuring autoantibodies is of clinical benefit (Bingley 2010).

1.5 The spectrum of Type 1 diabetes—LADA and late-onset Type 1 diabetes, 'Type 1.5' diabetes

As it is becoming clearer that the spectrum of diabetes, both Type 1 and Type 2, is broadening, further types are being defined. It is important to recognize that patients may be diagnosed (and managed) differently according to not only their phenotype at presentation, but also other factors—for example, to whom they present, for example paediatricians or adult endocrinologists.

The classical rapid symptomatic onset of Type 1 diabetes in white children is only one mode of presentation (see Chapter 2). An increasingly common presentation is in older people where symptoms are of more gradual onset, ketonuria, signifying insulin deficiency, may not be present, and therefore immediate insulin treatment is not necessary. Latent autoimmune diabetes of adults (LADA), first described in 1974 in relation to the discovery of ICA, is now an accepted, if still slightly controversial entity, defined as:

- Onset of non-insulin requiring diabetes in those aged 30 or over
- The presence of diabetes-associated autoantibodies (essentially GADA because of the methodological problems of measuring ICA,

Figure 1.1 Schematic representation of the course of Type 1 diabetes

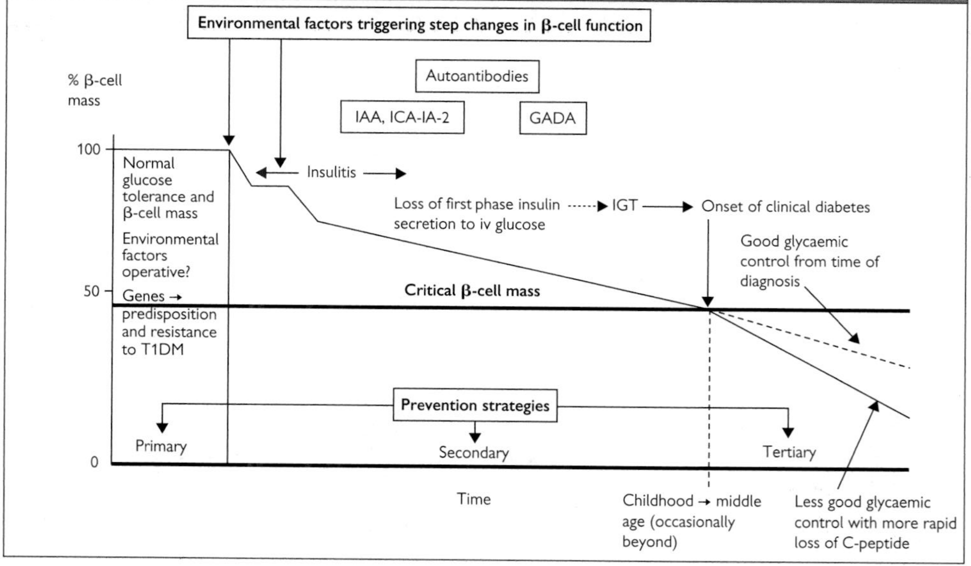

Environmental factors triggering step changes in β-cell function

% β-cell mass

100

50

0

Normal glucose tolerance and β-cell mass

Environmental factors operative?

Genes → predisposition and resistance to T1DM

Insulitis

Autoantibodies

IAA, ICA-IA-2

GADA

Loss of first phase insulin secretion to iv glucose ·····▶ IGT ──▶ Onset of clinical diabetes

Critical β-cell mass

Good glycaemic control from time of diagnosis

Less good glycaemic control with more rapid loss of C-peptide

Time

Prevention strategies

Primary

Secondary

Tertiary

Childhood → middle age (occasionally beyond)

and the low prevalence of IA-2 antibodies)—though their presence naturally does not distinguish LADA from Type 1 diabetes
• Interval from diagnosis to requiring insulin of >6 months (though this 'soft' criterion has been questioned; where GADA measurements are available, physicians tend to recommend starting insulin treatment much earlier).

The definition is therefore currently more useful in epidemiological studies than in clinical practice (Box 1.2). The converse approach may be valuable in defining the clinical characteristics of GADA-positive patients. For example, ~4% of patients recruited into the ADOPT study of newly diagnosed Type 2 Europeans and Americans were GADA-positive (Zinman et al. 2004), and in the similar population of newly diagnosed UK patients in the UKPDS, around 10% were GADA positive. However, in ADOPT, simple clinical criteria did not distinguish between GADA-positive and -negative patients (no gender differences, mean age 57 yrs, mean BMI 31 to 32). Fasting insulin levels and homeostasis model assessment of insulin resistance (HOMA-IR), a simple index of insulin resistance, were lower in GADA-positive than GADA-negative subjects, and not surprisingly, the National Cholesterol Education Program, Adult Treatment Panel III (NCEP ATP III) criteria for the metabolic syndrome were less prevalent.

Expanding the simple clinical criteria may be more useful. Two or more of the following were found to reliably identify LADA (Fourlanos et al. 2006):
• Age of onset <50 yrs
• Acute symptoms (<6 months)—osmotic, unintentional weight loss (but not infections or blurred vision)
• Personal history of autoimmune disease (autoimmune thyroid disease (AITD), rheumatoid)
• Family history of autoimmune disease (Type 1 diabetes, AITD, rheumatoid, coeliac disease) (Box 1.2).

LADA can be considered a relatively distinct form of autoimmune diabetes, but the increased clinical awareness of Type 1 diabetes, together with the availability of autoantibody tests, has reinforced the concept that autoimmune diabetes is a highly heterogeneous condition, existing along continua of at least four domains (Leslie et al. 2005):
• *Genetic susceptibility*, which is strong in childhood-onset Type 1 diabetes, but which weakens in LADA
• *Non-genetic influences*, broadly inverse to the genetic influences

Box 1.2 Case history: late-onset Type 1 diabetes with a long clinical presentation

A 45-yr-old male Caucasian had two episodes of abscesses of the skin of the neck (the first occurred 18 months before presentation). There had been gradual weight loss and osmotic symptoms for 1 yr. He had no family history of diabetes or autoimmune disease. On admission: weight 87 kg, 180 cm, BMI 26 (maximum previous weight not known). Blood glucose >30 mmol/L, normal venous bicarbonate. Urinalysis: 3+ ketonuria. A1C 10.0%. He was given an unsuccessful brief trial with a sulphonylurea, and then commenced on twice-daily fixed-mixture insulin. Four months later A1C 6.5% on total daily insulin dose of 34 units. After 7 months, A1C was again 10%, and with further weight loss of ~10 kg. He was converted to basal-bolus insulin, and 8 months later A1C was 8.4%.

- Anti-thyroid peroxidase (TPO) antibodies negative
- GADA positive

This case at presentation was clinically typical late-onset Type 1 diabetes with a long clinical prodrome. However, if the patient had been intercepted at the time of his first neck abscess, before significant weight loss, Type 2 diabetes would have been considered more likely. Doubt about future insulin dependence would have been resolved with a GADA measurement at the time, though it is unlikely he could have been successfully treated with oral agents for 6 months or more. Despite the very long presentation with markedly elevated A1C, he still maintained a honeymoon period for about 1 yr.

- *Diabetes-associated immune responses*, which also appear to be stronger in early-onset Type 1 diabetes (e.g. the presence of IAAs in children)
- *Metabolic abnormalities*: while insulin deficiency progressing at a variable rate is considered the endocrine hallmark of Type 1 diabetes, LADA is associated with insulin-resistance characteristics in many patients. In addition, there is data from the interventional European Nicotinamide Diabetes Intervention Trial (ENDIT) study that, by analogy with the 'accelerator hypothesis', insulin resistance in antibody-positive relatives accelerated progression to Type 1 diabetes, though only in those with advanced insulin deficiency (Bingley et al. 2008) (Figure 1.2).

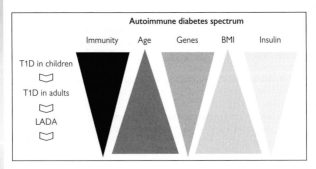

Figure 1.2 The spectrum of autoimmune diabetes. Five important continuously variable domains interact to produce the broadening modes of presentation of autoimmune diabetes. Courtesy of Prof. David Leslie.

1.6 **Autoimmune associations of Type 1 diabetes**

Organ-specific autoimmune diseases are very common in patients with Type 1 diabetes and their first-degree relatives. Two autoimmune polyglandular syndromes (APS) are recognized:

• Type I APS (autoimmune polyendocrinopathy, candidiasis, ectodermal dysplasia, APECED) consists of two or three of:
  • Mucocutaneous candidiasis with nail dystrophy
  • Hypoparathyroidism
  • Addison's disease.

Type 1 diabetes occurs in ~20%

• Type II APS. Much more common than APS-1, and usually found in HLA DR3/4-positive females. There is no universally accepted definition, but a combination of two autoimmune endocrine disorders is considered sufficient to make the diagnosis. Specific autoantibodies have been described in many of the conditions, and several are widespread enough to be considered for use in screening programmes (Table 1.1).

1.7 **Interventional trials in Type 1 diabetes**

Distinguish, where possible:

• Primary prevention: preventing autoimmunity
• Secondary prevention: preventing diabetes in subjects with known autoimmune predilection—those with multiple high-risk autoantibodies

- Tertiary prevention: reversal of the condition or preservation of C-peptide status immediately after clinical presentation.

Secondary and tertiary prevention trials have dominated the field so far, the latter capitalizing on the immediate post-diagnosis period where β-cell function is often partially preserved. Tertiary intervention studies in new-onset diabetes over the past 20 yrs included trials

Table 1.1 Autoimmune associations of Type 1 diabetes in adults

	Prevalence in Type 1 patients	Autoantibodies	Comments
Autoimmune thyroid disease (AITD)	Up to 30% (Hashimoto's thyroiditis), 1% (Graves' disease)	Anti-TPO Anti-TSH receptor	Associated with female gender and anti-TPO antibodies. 20-yr prevalence in Type 1 patients with anti-TPO antibodies ~80%
Coeliac disease	5%–10% (serological)	Tissue transglutaminase (anti-endomysial antibodies now obsolete)	~75% of subjects with positive serology have abnormal small intestinal biopsy findings. Risk of coeliac disease in Type 1 patients is probably increasing
Addison's disease	1%–2% (serological)	21-hydroxylase	Strongly associated with thyroid autoimmunity
Pernicious anaemia (PA)	~15%–20%	Parietal cell antibodies	6% prevalence of PA in Type 1 patients with AITD
Myasthenia gravis	Very rare	Anti-acetylcholine receptor antibodies	
Primary biliary cirrhosis		Anti-mitochondrial antibodies	
Others: alopecia, vitiligo, hypophysitis, autoimmune liver disease, juvenile rheumatoid arthritis			

of azathioprine, cyclosporine, and antithymocyte globulin with prednisolone; these proved to be either too toxic or ineffective. Other less toxic compounds, for example nicotinamide and Bacillus Calmette-Guérin (BCG), also showed no benefit. More recently, oral or parenteral insulin (the Diabetes Prevention Trial—Type 1) were ineffective, but the trial showed the practicality of screening large numbers of high-risk subjects (first-degree relatives). Further studies of intranasal and oral insulin preparations are continuing, and other candidate antigens, for example GAD65, heat shock peptide (hsp60, Diapep277, whose effects may be mediated through IL-10 or decreased autoantigen-specific T-cell proliferation), are being explored. Rituximab, an anti-CD20 monoclonal antibody, which may attenuate anti-islet T-cell activity, and mycophenolate with daclizumab, all agents in current use, are also being studied (Haller *et al.* 2007). Currently the most promising agent, and the one most likely to be licensed for clinical use, is otelixizumab, an aglycosylated chimeric/ humanized CD-3 antibody (ChAglyCD3). Given as a 6-day course within three months of diagnosis it preserved β-cell function better than placebo over 3 years and delayed the rise in insulin requirements over 4 years, with lower A1C measurements. DEFEND-2, a confirmatory phase 3 clinical trial is in progress. The anti-TNF-α agent etanercept given twice weekly successfully lowered A1C and increased C-peptide levels in newly-diagnosed paediatric patients over 6 months, and oral interferon-α better preserved C-peptide levels than placebo over a year. Results with these varied agents are encouraging, though concerns about long-term adverse effects may temper their use, especially in young children (Raskin and Mohan 2010). A new phase of primary prevention trials is attempting to manipulate putative environmental triggers, for example using different infant feeds, and there is one preliminary report of the benefits of autologous stem-cell transplantation.

References

Bingley PJ, Mahon JL, Gale EA, for the European Nicotinamide Diabetes Intervention Trial (ENDIT) Group (2008). Insulin resistance and progression to type 1 diabetes in the European Nicotinamide Diabetes Intervention Trial (ENDIT). *Diabetes Care*, **31**: 146–50. [PMID: 17959864]

Bingley PJ (2010). Clinical applications of diabetes antibody testing. *J Clin Endocrinol Metab*, **95**(1): 25–33. [PMID: 19875480]

Fourlanos S, Perry C, Stein MS, Stankovich J, Harrison LC, Colman PG (2006). A clinical screening tool identifies autoimmune diabetes in adults. *Diabetes Care*, **29**: 970–5. [PMID: 16644622]

Fourlanos S, Varney MD, Tait BD et al. (2008). The rising incidence of type 1 diabetes is accounted for by cases with lower-risk human leukocyte antigen genotypes. *Diabetes Care*, **31**: 1546–9. [PMID: 1644622]

Haller MA, Gottlieb PA, Schatz DA (2007). Type 1 diabetes intervention trials 2007: where are we and where are we going? *Curr Opin Endocrinol Diabetes Obes*, **14**: 283–7. [PMID: 17940453]

Harjutsalo V, Sjoberg L, Tuomilheto J (2008). Time trends in the incidence of type 1 diabetes in Finnish children: a cohort study. *Lancet*, **371**: 1777–82. [PMID: 18502302]

Harjustsalo V, Lammi N, Karvonen M, Groop PH (2010). Age of onset of type 1 diabetes in parents and recurrence risk in offspring. *Diabetes*, **59**: 210–4. [PMID: 19833881]

Leslie RD, Williams R, Pozzilli P (2006). Clinical Review: type 1 diabetes and latent autoimmune diabetes in adults: one end of the rainbow. *J Clin Endocrinol Metab*, **91**: 1654–9. [PMID: 14678821]

Mohr SB, Garland CF, Gorham ED, Garland FC (2008). The association between ultraviolet B irradiance, vitamin D status and incidence rates of type 1 diabetes in 51 regions worldwide. *Diabetologia*, **51**: 1391–8. [PMID: 18548227]

Raskin P, Mohan A (2010). Emerging treatments for the prevention of type 1 diabetes. *Expert Opin Emerg Drugs*, **15**:225–36. [PMID: 20384544]

Wilkin TJ (2008). Diabetes: 1 and 2, or one and the same? Progress with the accelerator hypothesis. *Pediatr Diabetes*, **9** (3 Pt 2): 23–32. [PMID: 18540866]

Zinman B, Kahn SE, Haffner SM, O'Neill MC, Heisa MA, Freed ML; ADOPT Study Group (2004). Phenotypic characteristics of GAD anti-body-positive recently diagnosed patients with type 2 diabetes in North America and Europe. *Diabetes*, **53**: 3193–200. [PMID: 15661950]

Further reading

Bliss M (2007). *The Discovery of Insulin (Twenty-fifth Anniversary Edition)*. Chicago University Press. ISBN: 978-0-22-605899-3.

Feudtner C (2003). *Bittersweet: Diabetes, Insulin, and the Transformation of Illness* (Studies in Social Medicine). The University of North Carolina Press. ISBN: 978-0-80-782791-8.

Tattersall R (2009). *Diabetes: The Biography* (Biographies of Disease). Oxford University Press. ISBN: 978-0-19-954136-2.

Chapter 2

Presentation and diabetic emergencies

Key points

- Presentation of Type 1 diabetes is highly variable, from fulminant (few days) to several years.
- Diabetic ketoacidosis (DKA) is a manifestation of β-cell failure, not of autoimmune diabetes, and can also occur in Type 2 diabetes.
- Partial recovery of β-cell function ('honeymoon') after diagnosis is common, and can be prolonged.
- Most newly presenting Type 1 patients can be managed as outpatients; relatively few now present with DKA.
- DKA fortunately now carries a very low mortality in developed health-care systems, but its management requires care, and very careful attention to fluid and electrolyte management.
- Severe hypoglycaemia is experienced annually by 10%–30% of Type 1 patients, though this figure may currently be lower. Follow-up of patients admitted to hospital with hypoglycaemia is as important as the emergency management.

2.1 Presentation

Type 1 (more precisely Type 1A—with positive autoantibodies) typically presents acutely in children and adolescents, symptoms being present for a variable period, usually around 3 to 4 weeks (range 2 to 10 weeks). Precipitate weight loss, osmotic symptoms of polyuria and polydipsia—sometimes insatiable thirst—and blurring of vision relating to osmotic changes in the lens are well known. As the spectrum of Type 1 diabetes changes, histories more typical of Type 2 diabetes occur frequently in older people with slower progression of β-cell failure that occasionally might be intermittent, for example osmotic symptoms that remit, recurrent staphylococcal skin infections and oral and genital candidal infections (see Case history in Chapter 1, Box 1.2). Neonatal and infant presentations are a major diagnostic challenge.

2.1.1 **Fulminant Type 1 diabetes**

A distinct sub-type of diabetes reported mostly in Japan, but also in South Korea and China, all countries where there is a very low background rate of Type 1 diabetes (Cho *et al.* 2007). It accounts for only ~7% of cases diagnosed as Type 1 diabetes in younger people, but ~20% to 30% of patients with onset at 18 yrs or older. Characteristically symptoms develop in people in their 20s and 30s over a very short period (days, rather than weeks, as in classical Type 1 diabetes). A viral precipitant is suspected. There may be weak HLA associations, but they are different from those seen in Type 1A diabetes. Glutamic acid decarboxylase antibodies (GADA) occur occasionally, but all other islet-associated antibodies are negative, and it is therefore classified as Type 1B diabetes. Patients present with C-peptide-negative ketoacidosis, and are permanently insulin requiring. Interestingly, pancreatic amylase and lipase are sometimes elevated, suggesting some exocrine involvement. The very rapid onset means that there is no antecedent hyperglycaemia, and in contrast with Type 1A diabetes, A1C is normal at presentation. The absence of C-peptide at diagnosis, again in contrast with Type 1A diabetes, results in a higher reported level of microvascular complications at 5 yrs than Type 1A diabetes, where in most cases there is residual β-cell function (Section 5.2.3).

2.2 **Remission ('honeymoon')**

After the onset of Type 1 diabetes, there is often a period of variable duration characterized by low insulin requirements (~0.3 to 0.5 U/kg/day, sometimes as low as 0.1 U/kg/day), good glycaemic control, and a low rate of hypoglycaemia. This 'honeymoon' period is one of partial spontaneous remission, the pathophysiology of which is not known. There are few systematic studies of this phase, but it is potentially important because it presents a window of opportunity for intervention to prevent or delay the final decline of β-cell function (see Section 1.7, Figure 1.1).

Between 30% and 70% of patients go into honeymoon within 1 to 3 months of diagnosis; it can last for up to 2 yrs in a small proportion of children, but duration is usually shorter, around 9 to 12 months. Better β-cell function predicts a longer honeymoon, so patients presenting either with DKA or long duration of symptoms—both surrogates for depleted β-cell function—have a shorter honeymoon. Much less is known about honeymoon in patients with later-onset Type 1 diabetes (or LADA), and there is an evident problem of definition, as many of these patients have relatively well-preserved β-cell function (Box 2.1).

> **Box 2.1 Case history—an approach in a patient with later-onset autoimmune diabetes**
>
> A Caucasian 38-yr-old man, not overweight, presented asymptomatically with diagnostic blood glucose levels in 2002. Insulin treatment was started, but even on very low doses (e.g. total 12 units/day) he was frequently hypoglycaemic. After a year insulin was withdrawn, and metformin 500 mg bd restored blood glucose levels to single figures but control was less good (A1C 6.7% compared with 6.1%), and he occasionally had trace ketonuria on routine testing. He was advised to take insulin with him on overseas trips. Islet-cell antibodies were negative 1 yr after diagnosis, GADA positive the following year. He remained on metformin for 2 yrs, but glycaemia thereafter deteriorated (A1C 8.7%). He was established on basal-bolus insulin, gained 5 kg in weight, and in mid-2007 the A1C was 7.8%.

2.3 Presentations of Type 1 diabetes not requiring hospitalization

General awareness of diabetes and its symptoms is increasing among the public, and Type 1 diabetes is often recognized by parents of children and adolescents, especially if there is a family history; older people with less acute or intermittent symptoms are likely to present later, and young children are still at high risk of presenting with DKA. However, overall, relatively small numbers of patients now present with DKA (20% to 30% in a Finnish study of children, decreasing between 1980 and 2000; Hekkala *et al.* 2007), and most can be safely managed in the ambulatory setting.

2.3.1 Characteristics of patients who can be managed initially as outpatients

- Ambulant
- Mild or moderate osmotic symptoms
- Ketosis (ketonuria/elevated capillary ketones) with no acidosis (normal venous bicarbonate).

Known Type 1 patients with these features may sometimes require admission—where there are underlying medical or social problems—but they can usually be managed by frequent visits to and contacts with the diabetes team. Newly diagnosed patients who are clinically well can nearly always be managed in this way, but substantial levels of clinical support are required:

- Diabetes educator for initial management and education
- Emergency telephone with access to diabetes educator
- Stable home circumstances with adequate family support.

2.4 Diabetic ketoacidosis (DKA)

2.4.1 Working biochemical definition (Kitabchi 2004)

- Arterial pH: 7.25 to 7.30 (mild), 7.00 to 7.24 (moderate), <7.0 (severe)
- Venous bicarbonate ≤18 mmol/L
- Urinary ketones ≥2+
- Blood glucose >14 mmol/L
- Distinguish DKA from:
  - Poorly controlled diabetes (elevated blood glucose, frequently >20 mmol/L), possibly with trace/1+ ketonuria
  - Ketosis—high blood glucose with ketonuria but no acidosis in an otherwise clinically well patient with known diabetes.

However, slavish adherence to definitions is not appropriate in the individual patient, and many will be intercepted at an early stage of DKA, when the strict biochemical criteria, especially bicarbonate, might not be met, though the clinical scenario is clear. Making these distinctions enables many patients to be managed in the ambulatory setting rather than being admitted.

2.4.2 Epidemiology

Mortality data on DKA is complex and difficult to interpret. Much of it relates to children up to age 17, and it is often difficult to separate out DKA in Type 2 diabetes, which carries a worse prognosis than in Type 1. Recent data from Denmark cites crude mortality rates of 2% in those under 70 (lower than the ~5% in earlier studies), 15% in those over 70. Surprisingly the same study found that the incidence of DKA had not fallen in this stable population with high-quality health care (Henriksen *et al.* 2007) and recent findings are similar for other countries, for example the UK. DKA is a significant public health problem and a major consumer of acute medical services and its incidence is rightly considered a reliable indicator of the quality of integrated care of patients with Type 1 diabetes. In contrast to country-wide data, many individual hospitals are now reporting only a handful of cases each year. Therefore, in localities where there is a high incidence, targeted avoidance schemes involving intensive education programmes and 24-h availability of community diabetes nurses for advice and early intervention have been shown to be effective.

2.5 Pathophysiology of DKA

2.5.1 Changes in counter-regulatory hormones

Complete insulin deficiency is uncommon. More often, omission of one or more doses of insulin, in combination with a condition increasing peripheral insulin resistance, drives patients into DKA. After experimental withdrawal of insulin in Type 1 patients, plasma glucagon levels rise rapidly, stimulating hepatic gluconeogenesis and glycogenolysis. Glucagon may also stimulate ketone body formation. Acidosis, caused by high ketone body levels, and dehydration stimulate release of other counter-regulatory hormones, including growth hormone, catecholamines, and cortisol, all catabolic hormones that are insulin antagonists (Figure 2.1).

2.5.2 Ketone bodies (Figure 2.2)

Insulin deficiency and excess catabolic hormone stimulate lipolysis in adipose tissue, resulting in breakdown of triglycerides to glycerol and non-esterified fatty acids. Glycerol is used as a substrate for gluconeogenesis in the liver and kidneys. The fatty acids are transported into hepatic mitochondria, where they undergo β-oxidation to acetocetate (AcAc), which is then converted into the other primary ketone bodies, β-hydroxybutyrate (β-OHB) and acetone. In DKA, the normal β-OHB:AcAc ratio of 1:1 can be as high as 6:1, and the normal β-OHB concentration of ~0.5 to 1.0 mmol/L up to 12 mmol/L. Acetone,

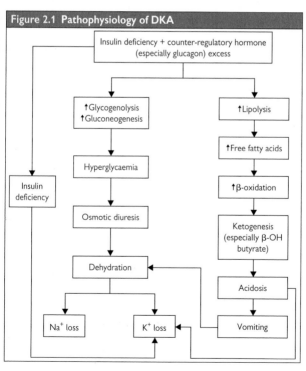

Figure 2.1 Pathophysiology of DKA

detected by standard urinary stick tests for ketones, is non-ionized, and therefore does not contribute to the metabolic acidosis, but some can detect it as a characteristic pear-drop smell on the breath of DKA patients. β-OHB is oxidized back to AcAc during correction of acidosis; urinary ketone measurements are therefore a poor indicator of success of treatment, as they may remain positive for some time after β-OHB has disappeared from the plasma. Quantitative capillary blood measurements of β-OHB using simple stick tests, similar to those for capillary blood glucose, are now available (MediSense Optium Meter [Abbott] using β-ketone electrodes). Because ketosis and its resolution are central to the management of DKA, these measurements should be used routinely.

2.5.3 DKA in Type 2 diabetes

Type 2 diabetes presenting as DKA is increasingly common. As in fulminant Type 1 diabetes, it is islet-antibody negative. It was first reported in obese African-Caribbean men in the mid-1990s, initially in the Flatbush area of Brooklyn, hence its occasional name 'Flatbush diabetes' (Banerji et al. 1994). In inner-city areas of the USA, 50% to

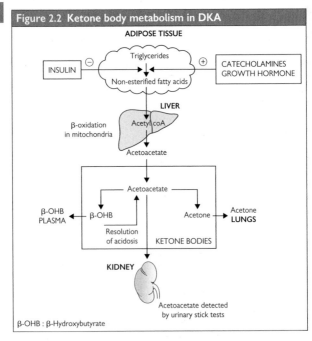

Figure 2.2 Ketone body metabolism in DKA

β-OHB : β-Hydroxybutyrate

60% of all cases of DKA are now associated with new-onset Type 2 diabetes, and it is a frequent presentation of diabetes in adolescents. It is now commonly seen in major cities in the UK in African and African-Caribbean people, predominantly men in early middle age (though its incidence will vary widely across Europe depending on patterns of immigration). So long as clinicians are familiar with the syndrome, the diagnosis is not difficult, though it is likely to become more so—classical Type 1 diabetes is not uncommon in black people in the UK, and the Flatbush presentation in adolescents, currently infrequent, may increase over the next few years. If acanthosis nigricans, the reliable cutaneous marker of insulin resistance, is present, then this is definitive evidence for Type 2 diabetes.

Attempts are now being made to classify all forms of diabetes presenting with DKA (resorting to the old-fashioned term for Type 1 diabetes of 'ketosis-prone diabetes') using GADA and baseline and glucagon-stimulated C-peptide secretion after full resolution of DKA ('Aβ' classification, Balasubramanyam *et al.* 2008). The classification may be of prognostic value—both for glycaemic control and future requirement for insulin—but C-peptide measurements are not usually available, and it does not help with the diagnosis of LADA, which by definition does not present with DKA.

In practical terms, the important point is that these patients presenting with DKA must have insulin treatment at least initially, but they invariably become non-insulin requiring. Characteristically, insulin doses fall rapidly over a few months, sometimes an even shorter period (low-dose twice-daily mixed insulin is appropriate, with careful hypoglycaemia education and frequent review), and in the long term most patients are managed on oral hypoglycaemic agents, sometimes diet alone, even if they do not lose weight. Recurrent DKA is rare but has been reported. The pathophysiology is not known.

2.6 **Management of DKA**

2.6.1 **Precipitating factors**

- Newly presenting Type 1 or Type 2 diabetes (10% to 20%)
- Infection: most commonly chest, urinary tract, or gastrointestinal (30% to 40%)
- Insulin errors or non-compliance (15% to 30%):
  - Most commonly failure to implement the 'sick day' rule not to stop insulin treatment if not eating ('no food, no insulin')
  - Technical errors (e.g. failure of insulin pump—now very uncommon—or fault with an insulin injection pen).
- Other causes:
  - 'Brittle diabetes', sometimes associated with occult eating disorders, most commonly in young women (see Section 7.8)

- Patients with advanced neuropathy and gastroparesis leading to recurrent vomiting
- Antipsychotic agents, for example clozapine and olanzapine, have been implicated
- Myocardial infarction, stroke, trauma.
- DKA is frequently associated with vomiting and missing insulin after taking alcohol, and cocaine use has been implicated in several studies as an independent risk factor for DKA and its recurrence (Nyenwe *et al.* 2007).

2.6.2 Clinical features (Table 2.1)

Table 2.1 Clinical features of DKA	
Symptoms	Signs
Osmotic: polydipsia, polyuria, weight loss, blurred vision	Dehydration
Malaise → drowsiness	Obtundation, coma—consider other causes, e.g. alcohol, drugs, meningitis, and CT scan-detectable causes such as stroke and head injury
Abdominal pain. Contributory factors: delayed gastric emptying acidosis → ileus ketosis rarely may mimic abdominal emergency Related to degree of acidosis, and alcohol and cocaine abuse	Hypotension and vasodilatation (acidosis) Ketones on breath (not everyone can detect them) Kussmaul respiration (air hunger)

2.6.3 Organizational matters

Use of protocols for DKA may reduce ICU and hospital stays, and also hasten biochemical resolution, but achieving uniform approaches to management is difficult because of the variability of presentation, and because there is a limited evidence base. This is shown by the wide variety of insulin and fluid regimens in use. Understanding the principles of treatment is therefore as important as remembering the details.

2.6.3.1 *ICU*

Criteria for admission to ICU vary widely: for example 30% of Danish hospitals routinely admit all DKA patients to ICU. The presence of any of the following should prompt a review by the ICU team:

- Impaired consciousness: these patients have the most severe biochemical disturbances, and young people are at risk for (or may already have) cerebral oedema
- Shock

- Co-existing surgical or severe medical illness
- Severe biochemical abnormalities, especially pH <7.0, amylase >3× upper limit of normal, rhabdomyolysis, severe hypophosphataemia (e.g. PO_4 <0.5 mmol/L).

2.6.4 **Investigations**

2.6.4.1 *Obligatory*

- *Urinalysis for ketones*, and where available quantitative capillary β-OHB. Document urinalysis in the conventional semi-quantitative way (−ve, trace, 1+→3+)
- *Capillary blood glucose and laboratory* venous plasma glucose, creatinine and electrolytes
- *Blood pH and bicarbonate*. Conventionally arterial blood gases are taken, but unless hypoxia is suspected, venous blood is adequate for both measurements (Kelly 2006)
- *Full blood count and CRP*. For unknown reasons, ketosis itself causes neutrophilia. A white blood count up to 25,000 is thought to be non-specific and not indicative of infection, but in clinical practice this would be a high count, and careful observation of temperature, clinical signs, and CRP are needed, always erring on the side of culture-and-treat. Clinical features of infection may be blunted by acidosis and neuropathy.

2.6.4.2 *According to clinical circumstances*

- ECG
- Chest X-ray
- *Cultures*: blood, urine, throat, cerebrospinal fluid (CSF), septic site (always quickly check the feet for painless infected ulcers)
- *Creatinine kinase*: rhabdomyolysis is described in DKA, and should be measured in patients with severe renal impairment, where alcohol excess is suspected, and if low phosphate is encountered on routine biochemical screening
- *Serum magnesium and phosphate* where there is severe metabolic disturbance
- *Amylase*: Values up to 3× the upper limit of the reference range are usually considered not clinically significant, but acute pancreatitis may rarely be associated with DKA. The non-specific abdominal pain associated with DKA may therefore be associated with similarly non-specifically elevated serum amylase. Salivary amylase, and reduced renal clearance are thought to be contributory factors.

2.6.5 **Management**

2.6.5.1 *Fluid replacement*

Total deficit is 5 to 8 L, to be replaced over 24 h—though a survey in Denmark found that most physicians plan to replace this volume over 8 h. Unless there is hypotension or shock, there is little justification for very rapid infusion of large quantities of fluid, especially in adolescents and older people, who run the risk of, respectively, cerebral oedema and heart failure.

Fluid replacement is with 0.9% ('normal') sodium chloride containing KCl 20 mmol/L, or 40 mmol/L if serum potassium is <3.5 mmol/L. Hartmann's solution (sodium lactate), increasingly used for volume replacement, should not be used. Lactate may be elevated in DKA, and can generate glucose (Dhatariya 2007). The first litre is usually given rapidly, followed by another litre over an hour, and the remainder over 24 h. However, take into account the effect of hyperglycaemia on serum sodium levels. Hyperglycaemia causes initial hyponatraemia through the osmotic effect of water moving out of cells, and this can be a significant effect with very high glucose levels. Since each mmol/L increase in glucose causes a true fall in serum sodium of ~0.44 mmol/L, a fall in serum sodium of ~13 mmol/L would be associated with a characteristic blood glucose at presentation of 30 mmol/L. Patients with normal initial serum sodium can, after rehydration, become markedly hypernatraemic (another reason always to be cautious with fluid replacement). Do the appropriate calculation, and consider the cautious use of 1 to 2 L hypotonic (0.45%, 'half normal') sodium chloride after initial rehydration with 0.9% sodium chloride. Note, in contrast, the severe hypertriglyceridaemia often seen in DKA does not have osmotic effects, and modern laboratory measurements are not affected by it.

2.6.5.2 *Insulin*

The primary reason for giving insulin in DKA is to suppress ketogenesis (this requires ~0.1 U/kg body weight/h, i.e. at least 6 U/h), as well as suppressing hepatic glucose output and stimulating peripheral utilization of glucose and ketone bodies. Insulin is usually now given by continuous intravenous infusion, though bolus intravenous insulin followed by intramuscular bolus injections is also used, for example in Denmark. The usual recommended initial insulin infusion rate of 6 U/h results in a rapid reduction in blood glucose over a few hours; once blood glucose is ≤15 mmol/L, intravenous glucose (usually 5%) is substituted for sodium chloride. At these blood glucose levels, and using a conventional variable insulin regimen ('sliding scale'), most patients will therefore receive only 1 to 4 U/h of insulin. This can result in:

• Delay in resolving ketosis because of low insulin doses
• Inadequate fluid replacement because sodium chloride infusion has been stopped.

10% glucose will cause more rapid resolution of ketosis than 5% glucose, as it permits higher rates of insulin infusion with a low risk of hypoglycaemia. Infuse 500 mL 4 to 6 hourly, maintaining insulin at ~6 U/h, and continue it until capillary β-OHB falls to <0.6 to 1.0 mmol/L. Many patients will require simultaneous infusion of sodium chloride (with potassium chloride) to fully correct fluid depletion (Figure 2.3).

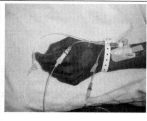
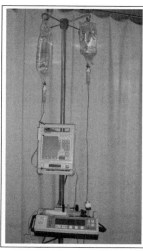

Figure 2.3 Fluid and insulin infusions in DKA. The syringe driver contains 50 mL 0.9% sodium chloride with 50 U soluble insulin, given at 6 U/h. At the same time 0.9% sodium chloride is being infused as volume replacement, and 10% glucose at ~125 mL/h

2.6.5.3 *Other biochemical measurements*

- *Creatinine and electrolytes*: measure at 4 and 8 h, thereafter according to clinical and biochemical state
- *Venous pH and bicarbonate*: monitor 2 hourly until acidosis is corrected
- *Potassium*: hypokalaemia, not hyperkalaemia, is the major risk: both insulin and rising pH drive potassium into cells
- *Bicarbonate*: not recommended unless there is severe acidosis and patient is gravely ill. These patients will require ICU care. Give 700 mL 1.2% sodium bicarbonate solution over 45 min, together with 20 mmol potassium chloride, and repeat until pH >7.0. In practice, bicarbonate is rarely required even in severely acidotic patients, once fluid and insulin have been given
- *Magnesium and phosphate* (see above): profoundly low serum phosphate is associated with acute alcoholic intoxication and may be a contributor to respiratory depression. Intravenous phosphates can easily be given, but again in an intensive care setting. No studies have confirmed benefit
- *Hyperchloraemic acidosis*: a transient non-anion gap hyperchloraemic acidosis may occur in patients given large

amounts of sodium chloride, as ketones are replaced by chloride. This can be a reason for apparent failure to correct acidosis in seriously ill patients. Replace or supplement with intravenous glucose as soon as possible

• *Lactate*: lactic acidosis (lactate ≥4 mmol/L), presumably caused by tissue hypoxia, may occur in up to 15% of cases of DKA (Sheikh-Ali *et al.* 2008)

• *Troponin*: between 5% and 25% of DKA patients have been reported to have elevated cardiac troponin I levels even in the absence of clinical cardiac symptoms or diagnosed myocardial infarction. Although subsequent non-invasive investigations (echocardiography and myocardial perfusion scan) have been negative, troponin positivity identifies patients with an approximately one- to fivefold increased risk of major cardiac events and mortality at 2 yrs (Al-Mallah *et al.* 2008).

2.6.6 **Management after the initial phase**
The initial set-piece management of DKA is usually managed without difficulty, but a smooth and efficient transition to early hospital discharge can be difficult. Involve the diabetes team as soon as possible. Once ketosis has resolved, renal biochemistry stabilized, and the patient is eating normally, the first dose of prandial insulin should be given 30 to 60 min before stopping the iv insulin infusion, on account of the very short effect of iv insulin.

2.6.6.1 *Establish the cause*
Review with a diabetes educator is critical. Many factors, especially in adolescents and young adults, may be operating. Typically, they are poor clinic attenders. Establish a definitive plan, with telephone contact in the period between discharge and a review appointment within a few days of discharge.

2.6.6.2 *Known Type 1 patients*
Re-establish and reinforce the previous insulin regimen unless, very unusually, it is clearly and directly responsible for the emergency. Discourage non-specialist teams from making unnecessary changes to insulin regimens, which may appear unfamiliar to them. Fine-tuning of insulin regimens is always best done in the ambulatory setting, once the patient has returned to more normal life.

2.6.6.3 *Newly diagnosed Type 1 patients*
There is controversy about the most appropriate insulin regimen on discharge for newly diagnosed patients, and practice varies. Factors to be taken into account are:
• Social and educational circumstances
• Patient motivation
• Ease of insulin administration

- Intensity of specialist follow-up
- The likelihood that many patients will move into honeymoon.

The Diabetes Control and Complications Trial (DCCT) found that intensive treatment (A1C <7%) can help sustain endogenous insulin secretion; however, the primary prevention cohort had a mean duration of 2 yrs, and there is no evidence that institution of intensive treatment immediately after diagnosis confers long-term benefit, and safety is the most important consideration. Many units therefore suggest starting with a twice-daily mixed insulin regimen (see Chapter 4) and move to multiple-dose insulin at an appropriate time after careful discussion with the individual, which may be at diagnosis in well-motivated patients. The total daily dose of insulin on discharge should be no more than ~0.5 U/kg/day, and may well fall substantially during honeymoon (see Section 2.2). The widespread practice of calculating a 24-h intravenous insulin requirement and using this as the basis for subsequent subcutaneous dosage is likely to overestimate requirements (and patients given high concentration glucose will inevitably have had high insulin requirements). For most patients, 20 to 40 U/day will be sufficient, divided conventionally as 2/3 and 1/3 given with breakfast and the evening meal, respectively, if using twice-daily mixed insulin, or 50% as basal insulin and the remainder as prandial insulin in a multiple-dose regimen (see Chapter 4).

2.7 Hypoglycaemia

This section deals with acute severe hypoglycaemia. For management of recurrent hypoglycaemia in the ambulatory setting, see Chapter 4. Every patient presenting with impaired consciousness to an emergency department must have a reliable measurement of blood glucose, and the result recorded. In Type 1 diabetes, aspirin, alcohol, and early pregnancy may be co-existing causes of hypoglycaemia. Factitious insulin administration is not unknown (elevated serum insulin, absent or near-absent C-peptide will confirm), and very rare causes, for example emerging hypocortisolaemia in associated Addison's disease, must be considered, but most cases of severe acute hypoglycaemia relate to the patients' insulin regimen and their lifestyle.

2.7.1 Epidemiology of severe hypoglycaemia in Type 1 diabetes

2.7.1.1 Definition (DCCT)

- Any event, including seizure or coma, requiring another person's assistance
- Blood glucose <2.8 mmol/L, or
- Symptoms reversed by oral carbohydrate, injected glucagon, or iv glucose.

In the DCCT, there was a direct, though non-linear relationship between severe hypoglycaemia and achieved A1C, and the rate was approximately twice as great in the intensively treated compared with the conventionally treated group. About 10% of Type 1 patients have an episode of severe hypoglycaemia each year, increasing to ~30% in intensively treated patients. Forty per cent of the DCCT/Epidemiology of Diabetes Interventions and Complications (EDIC) cohort had one or more hypoglycaemic coma or seizure, but only ~3% had recurrent severe hypoglycaemia. It is reassuring that an extensive cognitive evaluation of the DCCT cohort (mean follow-up 18 yrs, mean duration 24 yrs) demonstrated no appreciable psycho-motor impairment despite this high rate of severe hypoglycaemia. Nevertheless, ~6% of deaths during the study were hypoglycaemia-related, similar to the 2% to 4% reported elsewhere (DCCT/EDIC Research Group 2007), and the rate of severe hypoglycaemia was lower in DCCT than in more recent studies—motivation, education, and intensive monitoring are central to reducing severe hypoglycaemia.

2.7.2 Pathophysiology

The sequential defences against insulin-induced hypoglycaemia are shown in Figure 2.4, alongside their clinical correlates (Cryer 2002). In Type 1 diabetes, continuing excess of administered insulin causes plasma glucose to fall, and failure to increase hepatic and renal glucose production, while there is continuing glucose uptake in muscle and other insulin-sensitive tissues.

- Counter-regulation by glucagon secretion is impaired, for reasons that are not clear (probably an intra-islet defect—impaired glucagon responses can be demonstrated within a few years of diagnosis). Absence of glucagon is the major reason why patients with pancreatic diabetes are prone to severe hypoglycaemia (but develop less severe DKA)
- Impaired adrenaline counter-regulation is associated with hypoglycaemia-associated autonomic failure (HAAF), where symptomatic responses to hypoglycaemia occur at a lower blood glucose level after previous hypoglycaemia
- Cortisol and growth hormone responses occur only in prolonged hypoglycaemia, and are not critical for recovery from it.

Coma and seizures occur at glucose levels ~1 mmol/L, and if pro-longed, long-term brain damage is a real risk. However, in ambulatory clinical practice, patients may not only be fully conscious at these levels, but may also, superficially at least, appear to be behaving normally. The reasons for this huge variability in presentation and consequences of severe hypoglycaemia are not known (Figure 2.4).

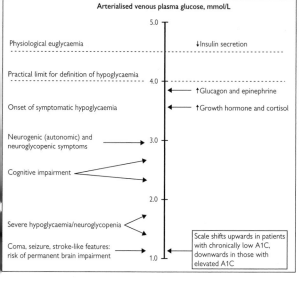

Figure 2.4 Physiological, clinical, and counter-regulatory responses to insulin-induced hypoglycaemia

Arterialised venous plasma glucose, mmol/L

Physiological euglycaemia — ↓Insulin secretion

Practical limit for definition of hypoglycaemia — 4.0

↑Glucagon and epinephrine

Onset of symptomatic hypoglycaemia — ↑Growth hormone and cortisol

Neurogenic (autonomic) and neuroglycopenic symptoms — 3.0

Cognitive impairment

Severe hypoglycaemia/neuroglycopenia

Coma, seizure, stroke-like features: risk of permanent brain impairment — 1.0

Scale shifts upwards in patients with chronically low A1C, downwards in those with elevated A1C

2.7.3 **Presentations**

Patients with severe hypoglycaemia admitted to emergency departments may not be known to have diabetes, and unusual presentations of hypoglycaemia should always be considered:

• Seizure

• Hemiparesis

• Aggressive (possibly criminal) behaviour

• 'He's been drinking, doctor'

• *Acute back pain*: opisthotonos or very rarely vertebral crush fracture caused by fitting

• *'Dead in bed'*: unexpected sudden death in young (<40 yrs) Type 1 patients, very likely associated with nocturnal hypoglycaemia and death possibly triggered by arrhythmia (Tattersall and Gill 1991). A post-mortem study from Australia confirms that sudden death in bed is still common, accounting for ~20% of deaths in young people under 40 reported to the coroner. This study found it was four times more common in males than females (Tu et al. 2008).

2.7.4 **Management**

Modern blood glucose meters are accurate in the normal and hypoglycaemic range, measuring as low as 0.6 to 1.1 mmol/L, and capillary blood glucose measurements are therefore reliable for diagnosis of hypoglycaemia.

2.7.4.1 *Oral glucose*

If swallow is intact, oral glucose is rapidly effective (15 to 20 g will raise blood glucose levels by 2 to 4 mmol/L within 20 to 45 min). If the airway or swallow is compromised, or conscious level depressed, do not use oral glucose or glucose gel. There is no evidence that 40% concentrated glucose gel is effective when applied to the buccal mucosa—parenteral treatment is needed. Glucose or sucrose, as liquid or solid, appear to be equally effective, but orange juice alone without added glucose is probably less effective. Clinical recovery may occur before blood glucose levels normalize—over-frequent capillary glucose testing is unnecessary.

2.7.4.2 *Glucagon*

Glucagon, 1 mg intramuscularly, is useful for management of hypoglycaemia by paramedics out of hospital, in hospital if venous access is difficult or delayed in a restless patient, and by partners and family members. The standard preparation is easy to make up by mixing the freeze-dried powder and diluent. It is usually effective within 20 min, but its effect is transient (~90 min) and must be supplemented by oral glucose as soon as possible. Patients with poor hepatic glycogen reserves (thin, malnourished, alcoholic, anorectic) may respond poorly. Intravenous injection can cause nausea and vomiting and prevent the patient taking oral carbohydrate, and the subcutaneous route may not be effective in a vasoconstricted patient.

2.7.4.3 *Intravenous glucose*

Preferred treatment in hospital and ambulances because of its immediate effect. Give 20 to 30 mL (10 to 15 g glucose) of 50% glucose by bolus injection into a large peripheral vein. Ensure effective venous access: extravasated concentrated glucose will cause skin necrosis, and even proper intravascular placement may cause phlebitis. Where available 20% glucose (50 to 75 mL) is less likely to cause these problems. Avoid forearm veins wherever possible in patients who are heading towards renal dialysis. Follow-up with a 10% glucose infusion if there is recurrent hypoglycaemia, for example related to a large dose of long-acting insulin. Maintain blood glucose ~10 mmol/L.

2.7.4.4 *Follow-up*

After emergency treatment and recovery, replenish hepatic glycogen stores with a substantial carbohydrate-containing snack. If there is full recovery, and blood glucose is >7 mmol/L within 1 h, admission is not necessary, but make firm arrangements for prompt follow-up by the diabetes team, especially if there is no obvious reason for the episode. Discharge within an hour is unwise, as it takes at least 45 min to recover full cerebral function. Always try to analyse the reason for the hypoglycaemia (take the history only after full recovery), and suggest substantial reductions (at least 10%) in the appropriate insulin doses, and more intensive glucose monitoring, pending a formal review. It would be wise to put any suggestions in writing.

2.7.4.5 *When to admit*

- Prolonged coma (>60 min) or residual neurological deficits after treatment, having confirmed normal blood glucose levels throughout the same period: consider postictal state, cerebral oedema, head injury, intracranial infection, bleed or infarction, or co-existing poisoning with drugs or alcohol. Get an urgent brain CT scan

- Patients who live on their own or with no facilities for close monitoring over the following 24 h

- Recurrent hypoglycaemia, despite adequate treatment, suggesting liver disease, or massive insulin overdose, intentional or otherwise.

References

Al-Mallah M, Zuberi O, Arida M, Kim HE (2008). Positive troponin in diabetic ketoacidosis without evident acute coronary syndrome predicts adverse cardiac events. *Clin Cardiol*, **31**: 67–71. [PMID: 18257021]

Balasubramanyam A, Nalini R, Hampe CS, Maldonado M (2008). Syndromes of ketosis-prone diabetes mellitus. *Endocr Rev*, **29**: 292–302. [PMID: 18292467]

Banerji MA, Chaiken RL, Huey H et al. (1994). GAD antibody negative NIDDM in adult black subjects with diabetic ketoacidosis and increased frequency of human leukocyte antigen DR3 and DR4. Flatbush diabetes. *Diabetes*, **43**: 741–5. [PMID: 8194658]

Cho YM, Kim JT, Ko SS et al. (2007). Fulminant type 1 diabetes in Korea: high prevalence among patients with adult-onset type 1 diabetes. *Diabetologia*, **50**: 2276–9. [PMID: 17724574]

Cryer PE (2002). Hypoglycaemia: the limiting factor in the glycaemic management of Type I and Type II diabetes. *Diabetologia*, **45**: 937–48. [PMID: 12136392]

Dhatariya KK (2007). Diabetic ketoacidosis. *BMJ*, **334**: 1284–5. [PMID: 17585123]

Diabetes Control and Complications Trial/Epidemiology of Diabetes Interventions and Complications (DCCT/EDIC) Study Research Group (2007). Long-term effects of diabetes and its treatment on cognitive function. *N Engl J Med*, **356**: 1842–52 [PMID: 17476010].

Hekkala A, Knip M, Veijola R (2007). Ketoacidosis at diagnosis of type 1 diabetes in children in northern Finland: temporal changes over 20 years. *Diabetes Care*, **30**: 861–6. [PMID: 17392547]

Henriksen OM, Røder ME, Prahl JB, Svendsen OL (2007). Diabetic ketoacidosis in Denmark: incidence and mortality estimated from public health registries. *Diabetes Res Clin Pract*, **76**: 51–6. [PMID: 16959363]

Kelly AM (2006). The case for venous rather than arterial blood gases in diabetic ketoacidosis. *Emerg Med Australas*, **18**: 64–7. [PMID: 16454777]

Nyenwe EA, Loganathan RS, Blum S et al. (2007). Active use of cocaine: an independent risk factor for recurrent diabetic ketoacidosis in a city hospital. *Endocr Pract*, **13**: 22–9. [PMID: 17360297]

Sheikh-Ali M, Karon BS, Basu A et al. (2008). Can serum β-hydroxyutyrate be used to diagnose diabetic ketoacidosis? *Diabetes Care*, **31**: 643–7. [PMID: 18184896]

Tattersall RB, Gill GV (1991). Unexplained deaths of type 1 patients. *Diabet Med*, **8**: 49–58. [PMID: 1826245]

Tu E, Twigg SM, Duflou J, Semsarian C (2008). Causes of death in young Australians with type 1 diabetes: a review of coronial postmortem examinations. *Med J Aust*, **188**: 699–702. [PMID: 18558891]

Further reading

Frier BM, Fisher BM (eds) (2007). *Hypoglycaemia in Clinical Diabetes*, 2nd edn. Wiley-Blackwell. ISBN: 978-0-47-001844-6.

Joint British Diabetes Societies Inpatient Care Group. The management of diabetic ketoacidosis in adults (March 2010). www.diabetes.nhs.uk

Kitabchi AE, Umpierrez GE, Miles JM, Fisher JN (2009). Hyperglycemic crises in adult patients with diabetes. *Diabetes Care*, **32**: 1335–43. [PMID: 19564476]

Wolfsdorf J, Glaser N, Sperling MA; American Diabetes Association (2006). Diabetic ketoacidosis in infants, children, and adolescents: a consensus statement from the American Diabetes Association. *Diabetes Care*, **29**: 1150–9. [PMID: 16644656]

Chapter 3

Inpatient management

3.1 Introduction

There will be very few Type 1 inpatients at any time, compared with the large number of Type 2 patients. However, they require even greater care when admitted for any reason. The intrinsic instability of blood glucose levels will be augmented by physical inactivity and intercurrent illness that will increase insulin resistance and insulin requirements; however, set against that, patients will often be eating less, usual meal patterns will be disturbed, and regrettably many hospitals still do not encourage self-care. Hypoglycaemia, especially during the night, is a particular problem. However, conversely ketosis can rapidly develop, especially in the ICU, in the post-operative setting, and when switching from intravenous to subcutaneous insulin treatment, and care must be taken to devise or modify insulin regimens to ensure adequate basal and postprandial insulinization. Continuous variable intravenous insulin infusions ('sliding scales' in UK usage) can generally achieve this, but at the cost of considerable discomfort and inconvenience for patients (intravenous access, often over a long period, and frequent capillary glucose testing), and increased nursing time. Extensive technical papers on the management of diabetes in hospital have been published, though inevitably the emphasis is usually on Type 2 diabetes (ACD/ADA Task Force 2004).

3.2 Insulin prescribing

This must be meticulous if patients are not self-administering; insulin prescribing accounts for 10% or more of inpatient prescribing errors.

- Take great care in writing prescriptions. For example, in the UK, 'Units' should be written out in full, or just the number if there is no space. Do not abbreviate to 'U', which can be misread as '0', or 'IU' (international units), which can be misread as '10'. Prandial insulin should be written in a way that ensures it is given precisely as the prescriber intends (e.g. '30 min before meals')
- Write prandial insulin both as clock time and in relation to meals, since meal times may vary.
- Premixed and short-acting insulins must be given at meal-times, not between meals or even at bedtime, a curiously frequent practice
- Prescribe insulin by brand name: generic insulin is not available. However, note that analogue insulins (see Chapter 4) have approved as well as brand names, and some patients refer to them in this way, especially glargine (Lantus®). In these cases, it is wise to prescribe using both names to avoid confusion
- Where the patient cannot recall the name of their insulin preparations, try to contact their primary care team, who will have a prescription record, or seek the advice of the inpatient diabetes team (who may know the patient, or will be able to suggest a temporary substitute preparation). Many insulin names, particularly older preparations, are similar-sounding and clinically significant confusion can occur.

3.3 Targets for inpatient glucose control in general medical and surgical patients

Observational studies have consistently linked high mean glucose levels with adverse cardiovascular and infective outcomes, but other than in the ICU setting, these have not been complemented by adequate prospective randomized studies. However, in many general medical conditions, and post-operatively, the observational evidence is strong, even for peak or isolated blood glucose levels >11 mmol/L largely associated with significant infections—urinary sepsis, pneumonia, and wound infections. Preprandial glucose levels between 5 and 8.3 mmol/L and postprandial levels consistently <10 mmol/L are therefore recommended, though these are very difficult to achieve in the acutely ill patient, and may not be beneficial (Inzucchi 2006).

Hypoglycaemia, often profound, is also very common in hospitalized patients, but patients may not have symptoms because of their underlying clinical state. Clinical teams must scrutinize capillary glucose records every day and make appropriate downward adjustments to insulin doses in response to evident patterns of hypoglycaemia: nocturnal hypoglycaemia is common, as is preprandial hypoglycaemia—the carbohydrate content of hospital meals is fixed, and patients may not have access to snacks.

3.3.1 **Management of unstable diabetes**

Management is complicated by wide variations in practice between institutions, and the difficulties and controversies surrounding subcutaneous 'sliding scale' insulin regimens still in widespread use in the USA. There are no specific guidelines for insulin management of Type 1 diabetes.

3.3.1.1 *Patients who are eating*

Depending on the medical or surgical problem, maintaining twice-daily biphasic insulin regimens may be satisfactory (with daily review of dosage requirements), but conversion to a basal-bolus regimen, with 40% to 50% of the total previous daily dose given as long-acting analogue or isophane/NPH insulin, will be more appropriate in many cases, because mealtimes are often different in hospital. Patients are frequently temporarily nil by mouth, placing them at risk of hypoglycaemia if the previous dose is given, and of insulin deficiency if it is not. The emphasis should be on basal insulin, targeting good fasting glucose levels.

Correction dose insulin can be given when unexpected high glucose levels occur and no scheduled insulin administration is planned (though it is not 'sliding scale' insulin), whereas in UK hospital practice, it is usually used for management of high nocturnal glucose levels. Small bolus doses (~4 U) of soluble or fast-acting analogue insulin are usually prescribed, but can lead to hypoglycaemia—or more commonly have a trivial effect. If given, they should not be prescribed at less than 3-h intervals to avoid overlap with the previous dose, and about one-half of any correction doses should be added to next day's long-acting insulin.

A small additional dose (e.g. 6 to 10 U) of isophane/NPH or long-acting analogue can be given for nocturnal hyperglycaemia, which will begin to act over the next 4 to 6 h, but prior blood glucose records must be consulted before prescribing, as some patients may run high glucose levels in the early part of the night, yet become normo- or even hypoglycaemic by the next morning. Great subtlety is required here, recognizing that isolated elevated blood glucose levels, for example >15 mmol/L, are common out of hospital, but are not detected because patients may not be testing in the late evening or during the night.

Sliding scale regimens in use in the USA refer to the use of pre-specified amounts of soluble insulin given in doses related to instantaneous blood glucose levels, regardless of whether the hyperglycaemia is related to meals. Basal insulin is not given. These regimens are regarded as unhelpful, because they are reactive and not proactive, and potentially hazardous because of the absence of basal insulin. They are rarely used in the UK.

3.3.1.2 *Nil by mouth patients*

When patients are not eating, a continuous variable intravenous insulin regimen (UK: sliding scale, USA: insulin drip) is usually effective. This co-infuses soluble (regular) insulin given by infusion pump in a 1 U/mL solution of 0.9% sodium chloride, together with intravenous 5% glucose infusion (e.g. 1 L 8 to 12 hourly), insulin infusion rates being adjusted according to capillary glucose measurements every 1 to 4 h, depending on the degree of glucose instability. Most patients will require intravenous potassium and daily monitoring of electrolytes—there is a risk of hyponatraemia with prolonged infusions of 5% glucose. Devising algorithms to ensure safety while coping with both absolute glucose measurements and changes over time is complex, and in the UK scales based on absolute measurements, which can be changed according to individual patient response, are usually used. Co-infuse sodium chloride if required. Where they are available, single-bag glucose–insulin–potassium (GIK) infusions are simple, safe, and effective.

3.4 Perioperative management

The aims of perioperative diabetes management are to avoid:
- Excess mortality and morbidity, especially through infection
- Severe hyperglycaemia
- Ketoacidosis
- Hypoglycaemia, during anaesthesia and recovery when consciousness may be impaired
- Iatrogenic problems, usually due to mismanagement of insulin, intravenous fluid regimens, and difficulties in correcting hyper- and hypoglycaemia
- Discontinuation of insulin at any time.

The stress response to anaesthesia, surgery, and pain is similar to DKA, starting with insulin insufficiency that may progress to complete deficiency if for any reason insulin is withheld during a period of intense catabolic stress.

3.4.1 Day-case and minimal-access surgery

Traditionally, Type 1 patients have been admitted to hospital before surgery for 'stabilization' of glucose levels. This is no longer necessary in many patients with good and stable glycaemic control and no evident complications, and with care, day-case surgery in Type 1 patients is feasible and safe. However, the metabolic response even to minimally invasive procedures is profound, and post-operative care must be meticulous:

- Fully assess patients for suitability for early home discharge, with adequate social support and where possible contact with the hospital diabetes team for advice on glycaemic management
- Ensure patients are first on a morning operating list
- Planning should be flexible—for example diabetes is a risk factor for conversion of laparoscopic to open cholecystectomy.

3.4.2 Pre-operative glycaemic control

Aim for good glycaemic control in patients for elective surgery, that is A1C ~7% or lower, though a balance must be struck between the urgency of surgery and the likely time needed to achieve this degree of control—and balancing improved surgical outcomes against possibly non-clinically significant improvements in A1C after a great deal of effort. Mean A1C in Type 1 patients is currently ~8% to 9%, implying estimated average glucose levels 10 to 12 mmol/L (see Chapter 9), that is values that carry an increased risk of deep sternal and leg infections in open heart surgery for coronary bypass. Cardiovascular events themselves increase as mean blood glucose levels increase, the relationship being non-linear and particularly striking at mean glucose levels >12.5 mmol/L that is A1C >9% (Furnary et al. 2003), though these studies have been conducted mostly in Type 2 patients. The current proposal, at least for open heart surgery, and probably justifiably by extension to all major general surgery, is to target (1) blood glucose levels consistently <8.3 mmol/L (150 mg/dL) and (2) three post-operative days of continuous intravenous insulin. Given intensive input and adequate time, for example 6 to 8 weeks, it should be possible to get suboptimally controlled patients at least temporarily into good control.

3.4.3 Practical management of perioperative glycaemic control

Many methods have been suggested, confirming a poor evidence base for this important aspect of surgical management:

- Wherever possible, Type 1 patients should be first on a morning operating list
- *For patients using a basal-bolus regimen*: give normal insulin with evening meal, and normal dose of long-acting insulin at 2200 (and in the morning if twice-daily basal insulin or morning once-daily)

- *Patients using twice-daily biphasic insulin*: give 1/3 to 2/3 of the total daily dose as an isophane or long-acting analogue at 2200
- *Intravenous insulin and glucose from early morning*: Probably the safest and most effective regimen is the single-bag GIK regimen (e.g. 500 mL 10% glucose + 10 mmol potassium chloride + 15 U soluble insulin, infused at 100 mL/h). This can safely be continued post-operatively. The regimen, also used in acute coronary syndromes (ACS, see below) and ITU, has become difficult to implement in the UK because of restrictions on adding drugs, especially potassium chloride, to bags of infusate, and unfortunately it has largely fallen out of use in the UK
- The more cumbersome dual infusion regimen, similar to that usually used in DKA, is now more commonly used (Figure 2.3). With either regimen, other post-operative fluids, for example Hartmann's solution or 0.9% sodium chloride, can be infused at the same time. Meticulous fluid balance and daily serum electrolyte measurements are needed (Gill 2003)
- *CSII*: where units and their anaesthetists have extensive experience of insulin pump (CSII) therapy (see Chapter 4), it can be successfully continued during surgery, disconnecting prandial boluses and infusing intravenous glucose with basal insulin delivered from the pump.

3.4.4 Post-operative management

This depends on the duration and type of surgery. In the UK continuous intravenous insulin is usually continued, while bolus subcutaneous and iv doses of insulin are more often used in the USA. An infusion of 5% glucose should be continued: iv fluids containing lactate can contribute to late hyperglycaemia. Urinary and capillary ketones should be monitored carefully. If ketosis develops, increased glucose concentrations and higher insulin infusion rates (as in DKA) can be used. Once the patient is eating, overlap subcutaneous and intravenous insulin by 30 to 60 min.

3.5 Co-morbidities relating to long-term complications of diabetes and surgery

3.5.1 Macrovascular complications and nephropathy

Younger patients are unlikely to have occult coronary artery disease, but it is more likely after 15 to 20 yrs, and in the presence of microvascular complications, especially proteinuria. The role of pre-operative non-invasive testing and which tests should be used to screen for occult coronary artery disease in Type 1 diabetes have not been established, though studies have repeatedly shown that Type 2 diabetes is an independent risk factor for post-operative morbidity and mortality. Exercise stress testing is likely to be of limited value; CT scanning for coronary artery calcification followed in patients with high calcium scores (e.g. >100 to 200; see Chapter 6) with stress echocardiography, where available, is likely to be valuable. Routine nuclear cardiology scans may be the best option in long-standing Type 1 diabetes with or without proteinuria. However, the most important point is for the whole clinical team to be aware of the possibility of coronary artery disease, even in relatively young people.

Fluid balance must be meticulous in patients with nephropathy, who are likely to have diastolic dysfunction; inevitably some patients with moderate or severe renal impairment will require short-term haemofiltration or dialysis. Patients with even mildly impaired renal function (e.g. CKD stage 3, eGFR 30 to 59 mL/min) may have epo-deficient anaemia.

3.5.2 Diabetic autonomic neuropathy

Diabetic autonomic neuropathy is the most neglected of the non-macrovascular complications in relation to surgery, yet probably the most important. Autonomic neuropathy contributes to cardiorespiratory arrest and post-operative hypotension (remember the possibility of unmasking Addison's disease in patients with unexplained intra-operative hypotension). Patients with any other significant microvascular complications, and those with symptomatic or diagnosed peripheral neuropathy (especially foot ulceration), should be regarded as being at risk for autonomic neuropathy even if it is not documented. Measure postural blood pressure changes and sinus arryhythmia (RR interval variation to deep breathing, see Chapter 5) and communicate the results to the anaesthetists. Recognize the rare fixed tachycardia of advanced autonomic neuropathy. Gastroparesis is particularly difficult to diagnose, but critically important in peri-operative vomiting and, rarely, in aspiration. Remember the association between Type 1 diabetes, eating disorders, and advanced neuropathic complications, especially in young women with long-standing poorly controlled diabetes.

3.5.3 Musculoskeletal abnormalities

Diabetic cheiroarthropathy (see Chapter 5) has been associated with difficulties in intubation; these patients are also likely to be at risk of autonomic neuropathy.

3.6 Intensive and coronary care

3.6.1 Intensive care

Even before publication of the work of van den Berghe *et al.* (2001), all Type 1 patients would inevitably require GIK infusions or variable insulin/glucose infusions in ICU. However, van den Berghe's team confirmed that maintaining consistently low blood glucose levels ~6 mmol/L with intensive insulin therapy conferred mortality and morbidity benefits, especially in those requiring longer surgical ICU stays. Benefits were similar for diabetic and non-diabetic patients, but separate results for Type 1 patients are not available. The follow-up study by the same group in medical rather than surgical ICU patients confirmed the morbidity but not the mortality benefit of similar intensive insulin treatment (van den Berghe et al. 2006). The need for vigilance over hypoglycaemia has been highlighted in non-diabetic septic ICU patients, where, using van den Berghe's insulin regime to deliver tight glycaemic control, a German study found a fourfold increased risk of severe hypoglycaemia (<2.2 mmol/L), an increased rate of serious adverse events, and a trend towards prolonged ICU stays. Further moderation of the enthusiasm for tight glucose control in ICU resulted from the NICE-SUGAR study (2009) which uncovered a significantly increased death rate. These risks may be even higher in Type 1 patients, especially those with longstanding diabetes with an increased risk of occult coronary artery disease (Brunkhorst et al. 2008). A clinically sensible balance must be struck. Continuous glucose monitoring may be a valuable technique in these patients in the future.

3.6.2 Coronary care

Even more controversy surrounds the benefits of tight glycaemic control in patients with ACS. The often-quoted DIGAMI study (Malmberg et al. 1997) studied predominantly Type 2 patients with ST segment elevation myocardial infarction (STEMI), and showed a reduction in mortality, but not of recurrent ischaemic events, with a regimen of intravenous insulin in hospital, and thereafter subcutaneous insulin. It has no relevance now that all patients with STEMI have primary angioplasty. All Type 1 patients admitted with any ACS should have as good acute control as possible (though there is no trial evidence), but the method for achieving this must be individualized—patients who are eating and previously in good control are probably best left on their usual subcutaneous insulin regimen with intensified blood glucose monitoring. Patients are rarely in a coronary care unit long enough to warrant a change from twice-daily to multiple-dose insulin therapy. Poorly controlled, acutely ill, or nil by mouth patients require GIK or equivalent intravenous regimen.

3.7 Glucocorticoid treatment

Glucocorticoid treatment at supraphysiological doses (i.e. prednisolone >7.5 mg daily or equivalent) will cause blood glucose levels to increase, and changes will be dramatic with acute high dosage treatments (e.g. prednisolone >20 mg daily, or 'neurological' doses of dexamethasone). In Type 1 patients, twice-daily insulin regimens will probably need changing to a basal-bolus regimen to accommodate the severe postprandial hyperglycaemia, and doses should be immediately increased by 25% to 50% as soon as steroid treatment starts. Because of the increased insulin resistance induced by glucocorticoids, hypoglycaemia is not likely, and persistent marked hyperglycaemia is troublesome. In patients with few insulin-resistant characteristics, insulin doses are likely to fall to usual levels rapidly after stopping the steroids. Even relatively trivial steroid doses, for example those used for intra-articular injection, may cause quite marked hyperglycaemia.

3.8 **Nutritional support**

Parenteral nutrition causes more severe hyperglycaemia than enteral nutrition, Where available, it is worth using diabetes-specific enteral feeds (low carbohydrate, high monounsaturated fatty acids, high fibre), as they cause less hyperglycaemia; other potential advantages of these formulations, for example on lipids, are less relevant in Type 1 patients. The evidence base for the benefit of specific insulin regimens is weak. Basal long-acting analogue insulin given at the start of a feed appears to be satisfactory, and carries a low risk of hypoglycaemia during periods when the feed is discontinued; however, basal insulin must always be continued, and 5% glucose infusion may be needed when feed is not running. If multiple feeds are given throughout the 24-h period, then high-mix insulin preparations (see Chapter 4) given at the start of each feed, two or three times daily, might help the post-'feed' hyperglycaemia. Monitor carefully and be prepared to increase doses each day. Ask the diabetes team for support and advice.

3.9 **Inpatient screening for diabetic complications**

Type 1 patients admitted with a diabetes emergency (DKA, hypoglycaemia) or for another, non-diabetic reason, must be reviewed by the diabetes team. They may well be young patients who have escaped regular review and have defaulted from hospital diabetes clinics. Wherever possible and appropriate for their clinical state, patients should have a systematic review (Box 3.1).

Box 3.1 Scheme for inpatient review of Type 1 patients

Clinical examination
- Weight and body mass index (BMI)
- Feet for peripheral vascular disease and neuropathy
- Arterial bruits
- Dilated fundoscopy, if not documented within the past 12 months

Laboratory tests
- A1C
- Fasting lipids
- Thyroid function
- Urinalysis
- Early morning albumin: creatinine ratio (although it may be falsely elevated by infection, fever, or severe hyperglycaemia, if normal, it will confirm absence of microalbuminuria; if grossly elevated, it is an alert to nephropathy and the need for further investigation)
- ECG

Other interventions
- Dietetic review
- Review with diabetes specialist nurse/educator—if possible identify areas in advance to be addressed:
  - Insulin regimen, especially if it was responsible for the admission
  - Equipment review: insulin pens, self-monitoring of blood glucose, monitoring equipment
  - Injection technique and injection sites
  - Social concerns: employment, school, driving status, family psychodynamics, alcohol, smoking, drugs.

References

ACE/ADA Task Force on Inpatient Diabetes (2006). American College of Endocrinology and American Diabetes Association consensus statement on inpatient diabetes and glycemic control. *Endocr Pract*, **12** (suppl 13): 4–13. [PMID: 17357258]

Brunkhorst FM, Engel C, Bloos F *et al.*; German Competence Network Sepsis (SepNet) (2008). Intensive insulin therapy and pentostarch resuscitation in severe sepsis. *N Engl J Med*, **358**: 125–39. [PMID: 18184958]

Furnary AP, Gao G, Grunkemeier GL *et al.* (2003). Continuous insulin infusion reduces mortality in patients with diabetes undergoing coronary artery bypass grafting. *J Thorac Cardiovasc Surg*, **125**: 1007–21. [PMID: 12771873]

Gill GV (2002). Surgery in diabetes mellitus patients. Chapter 41 in: *Textbook of Diabetes*, 3rd edn. Pickup JC, Williams G (eds). Wiley-Blackwell. ISBN: 978-0-63-205915-7.

Inzucchi SE (2006). Management of hyperglycemia in the hospital setting. *N Engl J Med*, **355**: 1903–11. [PMID: 17079764]

Malmberg K (1997). Prospective randomised study of intensive insulin treatment on long term survival after acute myocardial infarction in patients with diabetes mellitus. DIGAMI (Diabetes Mellitus, Insulin Glucose Infusion in Acute Myocardial Infarction) Study Group (1997). *Br Med J*, **314**: 1512–5. [PMID: 9169397]

NICE-SUGAR Study Investigators, Finfer S, Chittock DR, Su SY *et al.* (2009). Intensive versus conventional glucose control in criticall ill patients. *N Engl J Med*, **360**: 1283–97. [PMID: 19318384]

Van den Berghe G, Wouters P, Weekers F *et al.* (2001). Intensive insulin therapy in critically ill patients. *N Engl J Med*, **345**: 1359–67. [PMID: 11794168]

Van den Berghe G, Wilmer A, Hermans G *et al.* (2006). Intensive insulin therapy in the medical ICU. *N Engl J Med*, **354**: 449–61. [PMID: 16452557]

Further reading

Amiel SA, Alberti KGMM (2005). Diabetes and surgery. Chapter 15 in: *The Diabetes Mellitus Manual*, 6th edn. Inzucchi SE (ed). McGraw-Hill. ISBN: 978-0-07-143129-3.

Clement S, Braithwaite SS, Magee MF *et al.* (2004). Management of diabetes and hyperglycemia in hospitals. *Diabetes Care*, **27**: 553–91. [PMID: 14747243]

Joint British Diabetes Societies Inpatient Care Group. The hospital management of hypoglycaemia in adults with diabetes mellitus (March 2010). Diabetes.nhs.uk

National Diabetes Support Team (2008). Improving emergency and inpatient care for people with diabetes (diabetes.nhs.uk).

ThinkGlucose Campaign (NHS Institute for Innovation and Improvement) institute.nhs.uk/quality-and-value/think-glucose/

43

Chapter 4

Insulin treatment and transplantation

Key points

- The standard for basal and prandial insulin replacement is either multiple dose insulin (MDI) or continuous subcutaneous insulin infusion (CSII), both of which can give near-normoglycaemia (A1C ~6.5 to 7.0%).
- Careful implementation of MDI or CSII with a multidisciplinary team is probably more important to success than the specific types of insulin used.
- CSII can give remarkable results in some groups of patients.
- Only pancreas or islet transplantation can deliver true physiological insulin replacement.
- The results of pancreas and islet cell transplantation are continuously improving, and currently offer the only reliable technique for stabilizing and reversing microvascular, and possibly macrovascular complications.

4.1 Introduction

Though closed-loop systems are in active development, without islet or whole pancreas transplantation, full true physiological insulin replacement is not currently possible. While this is probably also true for other hormone replacements with physiologically less dramatic diurnal changes, for example, glucocorticoid replacement in Addison's disease, or even thyroxine replacement in hypothyroidism, the short-term and long-term clinical consequences of both hyper- and hypoglycaemia are wholly different. Even the dose ranges are completely different—around two-fold for other hormone replacements, but as great as 100-fold for insulin. The reasons for these differences are still not clear.

In the absence or near-absence of endogenous insulin, as in Type 1 diabetes, exogenous insulin replacement is a compromise. The nature and degree of that compromise will be different for every person with Type 1 diabetes. The evidence base for optimum regimens for insulin replacement is slender, and largely comprises detailed randomized controlled trials (RCTs) comparing one insulin formulation with another—or very slightly differing insulin regimens. The crude reported outcomes, for example changes in A1C, and categorical degrees of hypoglycaemia can only be used in the broadest way to inform discussions with patients about their unique insulin regimens. Meta-analyses and systematic reviews of insulin treatment in Type 1 diabetes have similar limitations. Finally, hypoglycaemia and the fear of it is still the factor that ultimately compromises the attainment of persistent normoglycaemia, and the increasing use of continuous glucose monitoring (CGM) confirms this in real life. CGM is a powerful analytical and educational tool, and will become an important therapeutic tool, but importantly for health-care professionals and patients alike, it consistently confirms the underlying instability of Type 1 diabetes using current insulin replacement techniques.

4.2 Physiological effects of absent insulin secretion and action in Type 1 diabetes

Total daily insulin secretion in a young insulin-sensitive non-diabetic person is ~25–40 units, of which about 50% is basal insulin secretion. In Type 1 diabetes, after eating, insulin secretion does not occur, while glucagon secretion is more or less maintained. If there is inadequate exogenous insulin replacement, endogenous glucose production is not suppressed, postprandial glycogen synthesis is decreased, and systemic glucose levels are high. Glucose disposal then occurs via non-insulin-mediated mechanisms, and glycosuria (Vella and Rizza 2003). Adequate insulin replacement normalizes these processes. Fat metabolism is also abnormal: insulin deficiency leads to increased lipolysis and elevated free fatty acid levels, which impair peripheral glucose uptake. Again, exogenous insulin tends to correct these abnormalities, but their dynamic complexity in the post-absorptive and postprandial states means that full correction is not possible with intermittent subcutaneous insulin. Figure 4.1(a) shows the astonishing stability of blood glucose levels in a non-diabetic subject in a 4-day CGM study—even mealtime excursions are barely perceptible; contrast this with Figure 4.1(b), a CGM study in a young Type 1 patient planning a pregnancy using a flexible basal-bolus regimen. There are postprandial peaks up to 11 mmol/L, but also quite long periods of hypoglycaemia, though A1C was consistently ~7.0%.

4.3 Insulin replacement

4.3.1 Basal insulin

Over many years, great pharmaceutical ingenuity has been deployed to prolong the action of native hexameric insulin, beginning with the

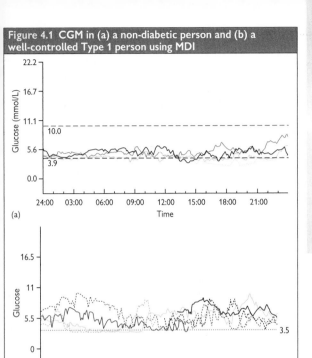

Figure 4.1 CGM in (a) a non-diabetic person and (b) a well-controlled Type 1 person using MDI

development of the prototype intermediate-acting insulin, neutral protamine Hagedorn (NPH; isophane insulin) introduced in 1950, as a combination with protamine and brought to neutral pH. Zinc further prolongs the action as lente (1953) and ultralente insulins, which are no longer generally available.

Two long-acting human insulin analogues, glargine and detemir, are now in widespread use. Glargine is injected as an acidic solution; crystals form at neutral pH, which are then slowly absorbed. Detemir self-associates into hexamers; absorption is delayed from the subcutaneous tissue and the circulation through the effect of the attached long-chain fatty acid, which in turn attaches to circulating albumin. Animal insulin preparations, both beef and pork, including very long-acting protamine zinc insulin (PZI) preparations, are still manufactured, though used by very small numbers of patients. While the progressive improvements in technology have certainly reduced the inter- and intraindividual variability of action of insulin (both long- and short-acting), variation in absorption from the subcutaneous tissue still remains a major problem. Significant factors contributing to this include physical activity, skin temperature, smoking, and lipohypertrophy (see Section 4.4).

4.3.2 Mealtime insulin (Figure 4.2)

Progressive shortening of the time of onset and offset of short-acting mealtime insulins has been achieved, first by changing from beef to highly purified monocomponent pork (1970s), then to biosynthetic human insulin (1980s), and finally to fast-acting human analogue preparations, of which there are currently three, the first of which, insulin lispro, was introduced in 1996. Various changes to pairs of amino acids result in a decreased tendency to form hexamers. Small numbers of patients use short-acting animal, mostly pork, insulin preparations. Currently available insulin preparations are shown in Table 4.1.

4.3.3 Human vs analogue insulins

There has been a longstanding controversy over the analogue insulins. Their use is restricted in certain countries, even in patients with Type 1 diabetes, where they are not considered to be cost-effective. RCTs, mostly non-inferiority studies, have compared them with synthetic human insulins (soluble/regular and NPH) and have reached the following broad conclusions.

4.3.3.1 *Fast-acting analogues compared with human soluble/regular insulin:*

- A1C is similar
- There are no differences in symptomatic, severe, and nocturnal hypoglycaemia rates
- They reduce postprandial hyperglycaemia to a greater degree than human soluble/regular insulin when given immediately before (though not when given after) meals.

4.3.3.2 *Long-acting analogues compared with NPH insulin:*

- Rather than being completely stable in their action ('peakless') they are better described as having a gentle onset and offset of action that persists for 22 to 24 h, compared with the definite peak action of NPH which occurs at ~4 to 6 h. There is continuing debate about the effective duration of action of glargine vs detemir. In Type 1 patients, increasing doses of detemir (e.g. 0.1 to 0.3 U/kg) show a rapidly lengthening duration of action from 7 to 14 h; at higher doses, more commonly used in clinical practice (e.g. >0.35 to 0.4 U/kg), duration of action is similar to that of glargine (22 to 24 h; Heise and Pieber 2007). Two studies have shown a small peak of action with glargine at 4 to 6 h clinically significantly reduce the incidence of nocturnal hypoglycaemia:
- Reduce fasting glucose levels

Table 4.1 Insulin preparations in use (UK)

Preparation	Manufacturer	Formulations	Approximate time course of action		Comments
			Onset	Peak	Duration	

Fast-acting analogue

Preparation	Manufacturer	Formulations	Onset	Peak	Duration	Comments
Insulin lispro (Humalog®)	Lilly	Cartridge, pen, vial				Best injected before meals, especially with high GI CHO meals. Glulisine has a faster onset of action than aspart.
Insulin aspart (NovoRapid®)	NovoNordisk	Cartridge, pen, vial	30 min	1 h	3–4 h	
Insulin glulisine (Apidra®)	Sanofi-Aventis	Cartridge, pen, vial				

Short-acting human (regular/soluble)

Humulin S®	Lilly	Cartridge, pen, vial				Slower onset with lower peak serum insulin levels than fast-acting analogues; similar time course of action after ~3 h. Detectable up to ~10 h after injection, compare 7–8 h for fast-acting analogues
Actrapid®	NovoNordisk	Vial	30 min	2–3 h	6–8 h	
Insuman® Rapid	Sanofi-Aventis	Cartridge, pen				

Intermediate-acting (NPH/isophane)

Humulin I®	Lilly	Cartridge, pen, vial				Marked clinical peak effect at 6–7 h, with tendency to hypoglycaemia. Most effectively used twice-daily
Insulatard®	NovoNordisk	Cartridge	2–4 h	6–7 h	12–14 h	
Insuman® Basal	Sanofi-Aventis	Cartridge, pen, vial				

Table 4.1 Contd

Preparation	Manufacturer	Formulations	Approximate time course of action			Comments
			Onset	Peak	Duration	
Biphasic mixtures (human)—soluble/NPH						
Humulin M3® (30/70)	Lilly	Cartridge, pen, vial				Mixtard® 30 withdrawn in UK (end 2010)
Mixtard® 30 (30/70)	NovoNordisk	Cartridge, pre-filled doser, vial	30 min–2 h	3–6 h	Up to 20–24 h	
Insuman® Comb 15, 25 & 50 (15/85, 25/75, 50/50)	Sanofi-Aventis	Cartridge (25, 50), pen (15, 25, 50), vial (25)				
Biphasic mixtures (analogue)						
Humalog® Mix 25 & Mix 50	Lilly	Cartridge, pen	30 min	1–4 h	12–16 h	Achieved glycaemic control similar to that with human biphasic insulin in Type 1 diabetes when used twice-daily. Can be used three times daily (with or without bedtime long-acting insulin)
NovoMix® 30	NovoNordisk	Cartridge, pen				
Long-acting analogue						
Insulin glargine (Lantus®)	Sanofi-Aventis	Cartridge, pen	2 h	4–6 h (plateau)	22–24 h	Once or twice daily administration (see text)
Insulin detemir (Levemir®)	NovoNordisk	Cartridge, pen	1–3 h		22–24 h	

Porcine insulin (and the very little-used beef insulin) is still manufactured in the UK (Wockhardt UK).

Porcine preparations are: neutral (soluble). isophane. and biohasic 30/70 (all available in cartridde and vial).

- Both are often better given twice-daily
- Reduce A1C, though the effect in RCTs is small (~0.2%)
- Detemir gives consistent small weight losses (~1 kg) while weight gain with glargine is similar to that with NPH. The reason for the weight loss is not clear, but it is greatest in the most overweight, and a significant mechanism may be its slight hepatoselectivity, resulting in lower effective peripheral insulinaemia, and therefore less peripheral lipogenesis (Hordern et al. 2005).

Studies have shown improvements in treatment satisfaction and quality of life-associated measures in Type 1 patients treated with analogue compared with human basal-bolus regimens (Ashwell et al. 2008). Nevertheless, individual patients' responses are highly varied, and there is still a place for human insulin preparations: for example, some patients prefer soluble insulin because of its longer action when meals are widely spaced. Basal insulin therapy with twice-daily NPH is still used widely and successfully, and may carry a lower risk of DKA (Korges et al. 2010). On the other hand, fast-acting analogues are ideally suited to patients who inject between main meals, and they are universally used in CSII.

4.3.4 Basal-bolus/Multiple daily injections (MDI)

The standard intensive insulin regimen by which all others in Type 1 diabetes are judged. Its principle is straightforward—to provide basal (background) insulin, especially during the night, and bolus short-acting insulin for meals. Its utility was confirmed in the Diabetes Control and Complications Trial (DCCT), where mean A1C values were only slightly higher than those using CSII (7.0% vs 6.8%). Counter-intuitively, severe hypoglycaemia rates with MDI are lower

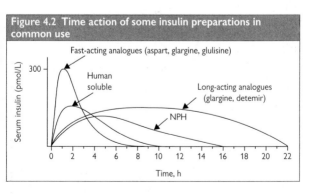

Figure 4.2 **Time action of some insulin preparations in common use**

in children and adolescents than adults, and meta-analysis found a strong linear association between hypoglycaemia and duration of diabetes—rates were ~4 to 5 times higher in people with duration >30 yr compared with <10 yr (Pickup and Sutton 2008).

While the physiological basis for MDI is sound, in practice, its successful implementation is complex, and requires:

- Frequent home blood glucose testing (see Section 9.1)
- An ability to adjust prandial doses in relation to carbohydrate intake, blood glucose levels, prior and anticipated physical activity, previous experience of hypoglycaemia, mental stress, and menstruation. This requires sophisticated continuing education, and specific programmes, for example Dose Adjustment For Normal Eating (DAFNE, UK and Australia—see Section 9.6.1)
- Frequent contact with a team experienced in intensive insulin treatment
- Use of the simplest, most portable, and robust physical devices for self-testing and injection
- Recognition of the considerable day-to-day and interindividual variability of insulin action, and that the use of MDI *per se* does not confer automatic glycaemic advantage.

Figure 4.3 shows some suggested initial strategies for distribution of both basal insulin (once or twice-daily NPH or long-acting analogue) and for mealtime rapid-acting insulin. However, the percentages of total daily doses conceal hugely variable absolute insulin doses: for example, a large-scale study in ~500 patients (mean age 35, diabetes duration 13 yrs) found that the average daily basal insulin dose was 0.37 U/kg (~28 U for a 75 kg person) and the total mealtime dose 0.46 U/kg (~35 U), while the dose range was 0.04 to 1.24 U/kg for basal insulin (3 to 93 U/day), and 0.02 to 1.67 U/kg for mealtime insulin (1.4 to 125 U/day; Bartley *et al.* 2008). These are useful indicative figures for introducing the concept of a wide range of doses compatible with good glycaemic control, especially to recently diagnosed patients, or those where a significant change in regimen is being discussed.

4.3.5 Practical points in MDI patients in suboptimal control

4.3.5.1 *Devising the management plan*

Full discussion with the patient, with particular emphasis on trends in glycaemic control, especially in relation to duration of diabetes, complications status, frequency of hypoglycaemia, and lifestyle reasons for current level of control, including an honest appraisal of adherence to injection regimen. Most patients will require a detailed dietetic review, possibly with a view to embarking on a structured educational programme (e.g. DAFNE) for meal-related adjustment of insulin doses. Some may require psychological help. Consider moving to CSII.

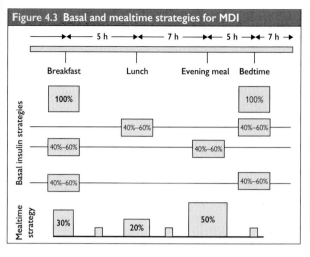

Figure 4.3 Basal and mealtime strategies for MDI

4.3.5.2 *Checklist of practical matters*

This should include:

- Type and dosage of insulin; technique for uniform mixing of insulin suspensions
- Injection sites (lipohypertrophy, overused sites, rarely lipoatrophy)
- Injection technique, including checking for malfunctioning insulin pen device, incompatibility between pen device and cartridge type, and between pen and needle. Ensure appropriate needle length for skin type and body build
- Check blood glucose testing technique and meter reliability.

4.3.5.3 *Establish diurnal patterns of glucose control*

Frequently, analysis of routine HBGM results will highlight patterns of hyper- and hypoglycaemia. If no pattern is apparent, consider performing a CGM study. This may uncover:

- *Nocturnal hypoglycaemia.* Very common, though less so with long-acting analogue insulin taken at bedtime. Encourage the patient to reduce bedtime long-acting insulin, especially when there has been prior physical activity or alcohol intake. If it persists while taking NPH, then a trial of a long-acting analogue would be appropriate. The correlate of overnight hypoglycaemia, the Somogyi effect ('rebound' fasting hyperglycaemia secondary to insulin resistance induced by counter-regulatory hormone secretion) appears to be uncommon.

- *Fasting hyperglycaemia*. Abolishing nocturnal hypoglycaemia may still not help fasting hyperglycaemia, or high variability of fasting glucose levels. Poorly controlled Type 1 diabetes (and puberty) is associated with the dawn phenomenon, exaggerated growth hormone surges in the early hours of the morning, leading to delayed insulin resistance and high fasting glucose levels (see Section 7.2). CSII, with increased basal rates in the latter part of the night, can correct this. (Declining insulin levels from an inadequate dose of long-acting bedtime insulin, which will give a similar glucose pattern, is uncommon, but easily correctable.) Where there is no evidence for nocturnal hypoglycaemia, and no evident dawn phenomenon, encourage slow upwards titration of bedtime long-acting insulin. In practice, modest dose increases (~10%–15%) are often associated with significantly improved control.

- *Postprandial hyperglycaemia*. This is difficult to manage. Even with fast-acting analogues (see Figure 4.1), it is clear from CGM studies that their peak action may not coincide with peak postprandial glucose levels. Simply increasing the dosage may therefore not help, and may increase the tendency to early postprandial hypoglycaemia. Some patients find the slower onset but extended action of soluble/regular insulin to be helpful for their particular eating patterns. A more rigorous approach to carbohydrate counting and flexible insulin dosing can be of real value, and modern insulin pumps have several ingenious strategies to help manage this problem (see Section 4.5).

- *Daytime hypoglycaemia*. Complex and highly variable. The prandial insulin preparation does not influence daytime hypoglycaemia rates, and therefore consideration of activity levels and meal composition is more important. Structured education programmes concentrating on dosage adjustment in response to varying carbohydrate content appear to be modestly successful in reducing daytime hypoglycaemia (see Section 9.6.1). Severe hypoglycaemia impairs symptomatic and counter-regulatory responses to subsequent hypoglycaemia (hypoglycaemia-associated autonomic failure; see Section 2.7.2) and although very difficult to achieve in practice, assiduous avoidance of hypoglycaemia for as little as 2 to 3 weeks can restore hypoglycaemia awareness—accompanied by increased adrenaline responses (Cranston *et al.* 1994; this initial study avoided hypoglycaemia for about 4 months). Optimized analogue therapy, CSII, and re-education on conventional insulin, all helped improve hypoglycaemia awareness over 6 months, although A1C improved only with optimized analogue treatment. Increasing use of real-time CGM over prolonged periods will probably play an important role here. Continual education about hypoglycaemia, its detection, and management, is crucial—too many Type 1 patients still believe that hypoglycaemia comprises only severe symptomatic hypoglycaemia, with impairment of consciousness as defined, for example, in the DCCT (see Section 2.7.1).

4.3.6 Biphasic mixtures

Widely considered inadequate treatment in Type 1 diabetes, they are nevertheless still in widespread use. They allow little mealtime flexibility during the working day, but are convenient. Few comparative studies have been performed, but glycaemic control is generally worse in patients using these insulin preparations (see Section 7.4.4). Not surprisingly, when used in a quasi-MDI way—for example, three times daily biphasic insulin aspart 30/70 with additional bedtime NPH as required to achieve good fasting levels—A1C levels were similar or slightly better than with a standard regimen of regular insulin and NPH, though achieved A1C levels were still suboptimal at 8.3% (Chen *et al.* 2006). Neither A1C nor hypoglycaemia rates are different with twice-daily biphasic analogue mixtures compared with biphasic human mixtures. In clinical practice, A1C levels of <8% are rarely achieved with twice-daily mixtures, though good adherence to this regimen may be preferable to a basal-bolus regimen in which mid-day (and possibly other) doses are omitted. While appealing, there is no evidence that high-mix insulins containing 50% fast-acting analogue (70% to 75% mixtures have been studied but are not in clinical use) are any better than twice-daily 30/70 mixtures. A variant widely used in paediatric and adolescent practice, especially where lunchtime injection is impracticable or not desired, is a biphasic mixture taken at breakfast, and a split evening dose—soluble or fast-acting analogue with the evening meal, and a long-acting analogue or NPH at bedtime. This is often used as an interim regimen between twice-daily biphasic mixture and a full basal-bolus regimen, but there is no evidence that control is better than with twice-daily insulin.

4.4 Cutaneous reactions to insulin

Allergic reactions to insulin occur less frequently with human and analogue insulins than with animal insulins, but they have been described with nearly all insulin preparations. Two major types are described:

- *Local skin reactions.* These can be either Type 1 (immediate hypersensitivity) or Type 4 (delayed hypersensitivity) reactions, and manifest as itchy, erythematous blotches, which can be troubling. Although complex desensitization protocols have been described, changing the insulin preparation (several trials may be needed) is usually successful. Very occasionally Type 1 reactions can be systemic and severe, and Type 3 reactions have also been described.

- *Lipodystrophies*. Lipoatrophy, probably an immune complex-mediated inflammatory lesion, is very rarely seen with human and analogue insulins, though it has been described in a few cases, even in CSII, where a local reaction to the delivery catheters might be responsible. Lipohypertrophy is still common with human insulin preparations, though it may not occur with analogues. After a while, injections into these sites cause less pain, but absorption may be erratic and delayed. Even where there is no clinical evidence of lipohypertrophy, absorption from persistently injected sites may be inconsistent and cause significant fluctuations in blood glucose levels—it is important to stress rotation of injection sites.

Insulin oedema, and even less commonly, insulin neuritis, is still occasionally encountered, even with analogue insulins, usually in older people with slow-onset Type 1 diabetes, presenting with high or very high A1C levels (>10%). The oedema usually affects the lower legs, but generalized fluid retention sometimes occurs, with facial oedema, and exertional dyspnoea. It remits spontaneously, but exclude the differential diagnoses of heart failure and nephrotic syndrome.

4.5 CSII (insulin pump)

First used at the end of the 1970s, insulin pump therapy for Type 1 diabetes is now standard treatment, though use varies between countries (e.g. from ~1% to 2% in the UK to ~25% in the USA). Specialist centres are using it with increasingly impressive results in children and adolescents, and some Scandinavian centres initiate CSII treatment from diagnosis in all patients, children and adults. In the DCCT A1C was ~0.3% lower in the CSII group compared with MDI, and in a meta-analysis mean A1C was 0.4% lower compared with MDI in adults. The effect seems to be at least as great in adolescents (Jeitler *et al.* 2008), and is consistent across different meta-analyses—for example, Pickup and Sutton (2008) found overall a difference of 0.62% in studies across all age groups, and a similar difference in studies comparing glargine-based MDI and CSII. This recent concordance in formal analyses strengthens the view that CSII is associated with meaningful glycaemic benefits compared with MDI. Total daily insulin doses are usually ~20% to 30% lower with CSII compared with MDI.

4.5.1 Acute complications

Overall hypoglycaemia rates with CSSI and MDI are similar, but severe hypoglycaemia is less frequent with CSII (Pickup and Sutton 2008). Since severe hypoglycaemia increases with diabetes duration, and also with A1C, CSII is likely to have the greatest beneficial effect in older people with the most severe hypoglycaemia on MDI.

Reported changes in diabetic ketoacidosis (DKA) rates with CSII are not consistent, and may be related to levels of expertise and support; DKA was increased in the relatively early DCCT compared with MDI, but there have been reports of reduced rates even in patients who would not be considered initially as suitable CSII candidates. With the advent of MDI using long-acting analogues, some patients may achieve A1C levels similar to those with CSII, but CSII will suit some patients better.

4.5.2 Technological considerations

This is an area of treatment in Type 1 diabetes where technological advances have been remarkable, beneficial, and have significantly improved safety. Basal continuous infusion of a rapid-acting analogue mimics physiological basal insulin, and all pumps in current use can be finely programmed to customize different basal rates, especially at night (e.g. to counteract the dawn phenomenon). Basal rates can easily be changed temporarily, for example during periods of inactivity, exercise and sports, menstrual cycles, and intercurrent illness. Spike boluses are given at mealtimes or to correct a high glucose level. Boluses can also be customized, for example as an extended (square wave) bolus for high fat or high protein meals, a combination bolus (immediate bolus combined with an extended bolus), or as a super-bolus (some or all of the basal rate for the following 2 to 3 h is borrowed in advance and added to the meal plus correction bolus, to bring down high glucose levels before a high GI meal).

Further refinements are continuously being introduced. Integrated software can calculate and suggest bolus doses, based on carbohydrate intake and prior glucose levels (bolus 'wizard'). Perhaps the most important recent innovation has been the integration of a CGM that sends glucose data wirelessly to the pump display. Despite the ~15 min lag time between blood and interstitial glucose measurements, these sensor-augmented pumps may soon be in routine use; one current device can be programmed to suspend insulin delivery temporarily in the face of impending pre-defined hypoglycaemia (see Section 9.1.1). A manual closed-loop system using a computer-generated algorithm has been shown to be effective and safe in avoiding overnight hypoglycaemia in children and adolescents aged 5 to 18 yrs; rapid developments in this critical field are expected over the next few years. (Hovorka et al. 2010). Sequential CGM studies in an individual changing from an analogue MDI regimen to CSII are shown in Figure 4.4.

4.5.3 Indications for CSII therapy in adults or children

These will vary between practitioners and centres, but consider CSII in the following circumstances:

- Recurrent hypoglycaemia, hypoglycaemia unawareness, or wide glycaemic fluctuations regardless of A1C; individuals prone to developing ketosis for apparently relatively trivial reasons

- Improvement in A1C: preconception, during pregnancy, early, potentially reversible, microvascular complications (background retinopathy, microalbuminuria)
- Difficulty in managing nocturnal glycaemia (hypoglycaemia or dawn phenomenon)
- Irregular shift patterns or frequent long-haul travellers
- Managing diabetes during exercise—fitness fans, competitive athletes.

In addition, in certain circumstances, patients requiring either very high (>200 U) or very low doses of insulin might be appropriate for CSII treatment. Although good compliance and high levels of motivation are usually considered mandatory, compliance may improve with CSII, and patients who are willing to have a try and may therefore become enthusiasts should be given an opportunity to trial CSII. CSII in adolescence is covered in Sections 7.4.3 and 7.4.4.

4.6 Alternative routes of insulin administration

After many years in development, the first inhaled (prandial) insulin preparation (Exubera®, Pfizer) was introduced in the UK in 2006. It was withdrawn in late 2007, few patients having used it. Reasons for its limited success include inconvenience of the delivery device, the complex dosing, the need for pulmonary function testing, limitations of use in people with chronic lung disease and in smokers, and its high cost. There were continuing concerns about adverse pulmonary effects. However, many practitioners reported good outcomes in truly needle-phobic patients, or those with severe behavioural problems that made injections difficult for carers. On the back of this disappointing experience, other inhaled insulin preparations in late-stage development may not be introduced. Alternative administration routes are being explored, including oral insulin, designed for buccal or intestinal absorption—the former may act quickly enough to be used as prandial insulin.

4.7 Adjuvant blood glucose lowering treatments

4.7.1 Metformin

The insulin-sensitizer metformin is widely used off-license in Type 1 patients, especially those with perceived 'insulin resistance' characteristics such as high daily insulin use and obesity (see Section 6.7 for further discussion of the impact of insulin resistance/metabolic syndrome on Type 1 diabetes and its complications). However, clinical

Figure 4.4 Sequential CGM studies (mmol/L) in a patient changing from MDI to CSII

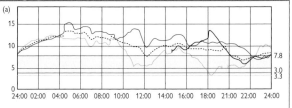

(a)

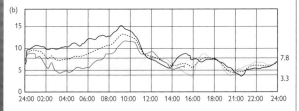

(b)

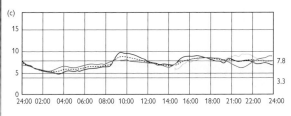

(c)

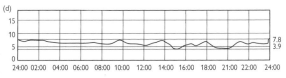

(d)

(a)–(c) CGM tracings (3 days + average [dotted line]—Medtronic Guardian Real-Time®
(d) single day—Medtronic Continuous Glucose Monitor Gold®)
26-yr-old male, 89 kg, BMI 31, frequent hypoglycaemia and fear of hypoglycaemia, preventing exercise.
(a) Basal insulin Lantus® 32 U, prandial insulin NovoRapid® 12:16:14. Total daily dose 74 U. Rising blood glucose levels in early morning (dawn phenomenon). (b) Three weeks after starting intensive education, still on MDI. Improved daytime glucose control, dawn phenomenon still present. (c) Three weeks after starting CSII (Medtronic Paradigm 722). Total daily dose 52 U (30% reduction). (d) Six weeks after starting CSII: near-normoglycaemia, total daily dose 45 U (40% reduction). No hypoglycaemia, overall weight loss 3.2 kg. Courtesy of Laila King and London Medical.

trial evidence supporting its use in Type 1 patients is slender. Studies give inconsistent results, but small short-term reductions in A1C (e.g. 0.5% to 0.8%), BMI, and insulin dose may occur (Moon *et al*. 2007). However, these may not be clinically significant effects. There is always concern about lactic acidosis, although it has not been reported in this situation (but see Chapter 2). Adding metformin may be justified where there is a separate, clear cut, indication, for example definite polycystic ovarian syndrome, common in Type 1 diabetes.

4.7.2 **Pramlintide (synthetic amylin)**

Amylin is a β-cell peptide hormone, co-located with insulin, and co-secreted with it in response to nutrient intake in the postprandial period. It is therefore absent in Type 1 diabetes. It is not considered an incretin since it is not gut-derived. It has three principal actions that decrease postprandial glucose excursions:

- Reduces gastric emptying (which may be accelerated in Type 1 diabetes, possibly due to amylin deficiency) of both solids and liquids
- Suppresses postprandial hyperglucagonaemia
- Promotes satiety, independent of its frequent side effect of nausea.

It is given by subcutaneous injection (preloaded pens are available) at a site remote from that used for the prandial insulin dose.

Placebo-controlled RCTs have shown:

- A1C reduction ~0.3% to 0.4% at doses of 30 to 60 µg, maintained in open-label studies for up to 2 yrs, with small reductions in total daily prandial insulin dose
- Sustained placebo-subtracted weight loss ~1.5 kg.

Severe hypoglycaemia and nausea can be reduced by careful dose titration, starting at 15 µg, and by reducing prandial insulin doses by up to 50% in the first month of treatment. Pramlintide is useful in patients already on intensive insulin treatment (MDI or CSII) and nearing target A1C, where postprandial hyperglycaemia is prominent (Pullman *et al*. 2006). It is so far not available in Europe.

Exendin-4 has similar extra-pancreatic effects to pramlintide in C-peptide-negative Type 1 patients, though its synthetic derivative (exenatide) is not licensed in Type 1 diabetes.

4.8 **Islet and pancreas transplantation**

4.8.1 **Islet transplantation**

Islet autografts in patients requiring pancreatectomy for painful chronic pancreatitis were first performed in 1980, and in the same year the first allogeneic islet transplantation was reported. The patient achieved insulin independence for 9 months with normal glucose levels. Thereafter, procedures were performed intermittently, but worldwide interest revived in 2000 when Shapiro's team in Edmonton,

Canada, used a novel islet isolation technique, and a new low-dose, non-steroid immunosuppressive regimen of daclizumab, tacrolimus, and sirolimus. Islets from multiple donors were injected directly into the portal vein. Seven patients were initially reported—all became insulin independent, with normal glucose and A1C levels. Between 2000 and 2006, ~550 islet transplantations were performed in about 40 institutions worldwide.

An international multicentre study of 36 patients transplanted using the standardized Edmonton protocol reported in 2006. Up to three islet infusions per patient were permitted, provided there was still residual islet function after the preceding infusion. The clinical characteristics of the patients are shown in Box 4.1. One year after the final infusion, about one-half (44%) were insulin independent with A1C <6.5%; about one-quarter (28%) had partial graft function (some preserved C-peptide secretion, but required insulin or had A1C >6.5%); the remaining one-quarter (28%) had complete graft loss (Shapiro et al. 2006).

At first sight these results are disappointing. However, there was considerable variability in results from different centres, and those performing more procedures were more successful in achieving insulin independence. While the majority of patients lost insulin independence, persistent islet function is important in maintaining glycaemic stability, and preventing severe hypoglycaemia in those patients transplanted for this indication. Even when there has been graft failure, hypoglycaemia awareness also seems to be reliably restored. The numbers transplanted are low, follow-up so far is not very long, and there is therefore no evidence yet of benefit of islet transplantation on microvascular complications.

Despite the low-dose immunosuppressive regimen, both tacrolimus and sirolimus have significant side effects, for example, drug-related toxicity (mouth ulceration, anaemia, and leucopenia), and renal and islet cell toxicity—renal function deteriorated in some patients.

The technique is still relatively new, and refinements will continue to improve outcome and reduce side effects. For example, in 2005 promising preliminary results were reported with single-donor marginal-dose islet transplantation (around two-thirds number of islets/kg compared with the Edmonton procedure) and using a different anti-rejection protocol, though patients using >40 U insulin/day were excluded.

Only 7% of the ~2000 patients initially screened for the international study of the Edmonton protocol fulfilled the screening criteria, and fewer than 2% of those originally referred were finally transplanted. While these are important data to discuss with prospective subjects, the procedure should always be borne in mind, and referrals made to appropriate local or regional centres. Indications vary, but are broadly outlined in Box 4.2.

> **Box 4.1 Characteristics of patients in the Edmonton International Study (Shapiro et al. 2006)**
> - Mean age: 41 yrs (range 23–59)
> - Mean duration: 27 yrs (range 11–51)
> - Mean BMI 22: (range 19–26)
> - Median insulin requirement: 0.52 U/kg/day
> - Median number of islet infusions: 2

> **Box 4.2 Eligibility and exclusion criteria for islet transplantation (Edmonton/*King's; Srinavasan et al. 2007)**
> **Eligibility criteria**
> - Type 1 diabetes, duration >5 yrs
> - Age 18–65
> - Undetectable C-peptide levels
> - *Primary indication*: recurrent severe hypoglycaemia >1 yr duration, ≥2 episodes per 6 months, including hypoglycaemia unawareness or severe glycaemic liability
> - *Secondary indication*: progressive microvascular complications: retinopathy, worsening albuminuria within the microalbuminuric range (<300 mg/24 h), worsening painful neuropathy
> - Failure of all attempts to optimize intensive insulin therapy and glycaemic monitoring, and where appropriate *management of hypertension and ACE inhibitor therapy
> **Major exclusion criteria**
> - BMI >26; weight >70 kg (women), >75 kg (men); *BMI ≥28
> - Insulin requirement >0.7 U/kg/day
> - Serum creatinine >135 µmol/L or *creatinine clearance <85 mL/min/1.73 m^2

4.8.2 Whole pancreas transplantation

First performed in a Type 1 patient in 1966, whole pancreas transplantation has a much longer track record than islet transplantation, and when successful can result in long-term normoglycaemia and insulin independence. More than 20,000 have been performed, about 80% in the USA (Larsen 2004). The centre performing the largest number of procedures, the University of Minnesota, reports a 5-yr patient survival of 90%, and a 1-yr pancreas graft survival rate of 70%.

Pancreas transplantation is a group of procedures usually, but not always, performed in patients in end-stage renal disease:
- Pancreas-alone transplant (~5% of procedures)
- Pancreas-after-kidney transplant (PAK, ~10% to 20%)
- Simultaneous pancreas kidney transplant (SPK, ~80%).

The high proportion of SPK reflects the fact that patient and kidney graft survival is at least as high as that of kidney-alone transplants, and patient survival consistently higher, possibly related to the normoglycaemia. Pancreas-alone transplants are usually carried out in younger patients with frequent severe acute complications (hypoglycaemia and DKA). PAK is increasingly performed; so long as renal function is stable after renal transplantation, the outcomes for subsequent pancreas transplantation are not different whether performed early (<4 months) or later (>4 months).

The same donor is usually used in simultaneous transplantation. Surgical techniques for pancreas transplantation are continually being refined: currently, enteric drainage of the exocrine pancreatic duct is favoured over bladder drainage, and although avoiding systemic hyperinsulinaemia by creating a portal venous rather than a systemic anastomosis may be metabolically preferable, there is no difference in pancreas graft survival. Normoglycaemia, defined as non-diabetic A1C values (<5%), restoration of the acute insulin response, and normal oscillations of insulin secretion can be maintained for up to 20 yrs after successful transplantation (Robertson et al. 1999).

Any pancreatic transplantation procedure is a major undertaking. Patients require much more extensive pre-operative work-up compared with islet-cell recipients, and post-operative follow-up is physically, psychologically, and emotionally taxing. Nevertheless, in patients about to undergo renal transplantation, pancreas transplantation should also be considered, and discussion opened with the patient, though often it is not.

4.8.2.1 *Effect of pancreas transplantation on diabetic complications*

Glucagon and symptomatic responses to hypoglycaemia markedly improve after transplantation; adrenaline and growth hormone responses improve but do not normalize. Remarkably, there is histological resolution of the lesions of diabetic nephropathy in native kidneys 5 to 10 yrs after successful transplantation. There is less conclusive evidence for improvements in retinopathy—many transplant patients have advanced diabetic eye disease, and already had undergone extensive laser treatment and vitrectomy. Most studies report stabilization of retinopathy after a few years, but there is still the risk of transient deterioration in retinopathy with rapid restoration of normoglycaemia after transplantation. Progression of cataracts, especially in steroid-treated patients, is common. Peripheral neuropathy improves after 4 to 8 yrs, especially after SPK, but autonomic neuropathy is notoriously resistant to improvement with prolonged normoglycaemia, and there are inconsistent changes up to 10 yrs. Populations studied are too small to show any improvements in cardiovascular event rates, but intermediate measures (e.g. quantitative coronary angiography, carotid intima–media thickness) improve within a few years. Foot infections and amputations remain common. Quality of life probably improves overall, but is moderated by expectation and success of the procedure, and post-operative complications.

References

Ashwell SG, Bradley C, Stephens JW, Witthaus E, Home PD (2008). Treatment satisfaction and quality of life with insulin glargine plus insulin lispro compared with NPH insulin plus unmodified human insulin in people with Type 1 diabetes. *Diabetes Care*, **31**: 1112–7. [PMID: 18339977]

Bartley PC, Bogoev M, Larsen J, Philotheou A (2008). Long-term efficacy and safety of insulin detemir compared to Neutral Protamine Hagedorn insulin in patients with Type 1 diabetes using treat-to-target basal-bolus regimen with insulin aspart at meals: a 2-year, randomized, controlled trial. *Diabet Med*, **25**: 442–9. [PMID: 18387078]

Chen JW, Lauritzen T, Bojesen A *et al.* (2006). Multiple mealtime administration of biphasic insulin aspart 30 versus traditional basal-bolus human insulin treatment in patients with type 1 diabetes. *Diabetes Obes Metab*, **8**: 682–9. [PMID: 17026493]

Cranston I, Lomas J, Maran A, Macdonald I, Amiel SA (1994). Restoration of hypoglycaemia awareness in patients with long-duration insulin-dependent diabetes. *Lancet*, **30**: 283–7. [PMID: 7914259]

Heise T, Pieber TR (2007). Towards peakless, reproducible and long-acting insulins. An assessment of the basal analogues based on iso-glycaemic clamp studies. *Diabetes Obes Metab*, **9**: 648–59. [PMID: 17645556]

Hordern SV, Wright JE, Umpleby AM, Shojaee-Moradie F, Amiss J, Russell-Jones DL (2005). Comparison of the effects on glucose and lipid metabolism of equipotent doses of insulin detemir and NPH insulin with a 16-h euglycaemic clamp. *Diabetologia*, **48**: 420–6. [PMID: 15729576]

Hovorka R, Allen JM, Elleri D *et al.* (2010). Manual closed-loop insulin delivery in children and adolescents with type 1 diabetes: a phase 2 randomised crossover trial. *Lancet*, **375**: 743–51. [PMID: 20138357].

Jeitler K, Horvath K, Berghold A *et al.* (2008). Continuous subcutaneous insulin infusion versus multiple daily insulin injections in patients with diabetes mellitus: systematic review and meta-analysis. *Diabetologia*, **51**: 941–51. [PMID: 18351320]

Karges B, Kapellen T, Neu A *et al.*; for the DPV initiative and the German BMBF Competence Network Diabetes mellitus (2010). Long-acting insulin analogs and the risk of diabetic ketoacidosis in children and adolescents with type 1 diabetes. *Diabetes Care*, **33**. [PMID: 20185733]

Larsen JL (2004). Pancreas transplantation: indications and consequences. *Endocr Rev*, **25**: 919–46. [PMID: 15583028]

Moon RJ, Bascombe LA, Holt RI (2007). The addition of metformin in type 1 diabetes improves insulin sensitivity, diabetic control, body composition and patient well-being. *Diabetes Obes Metab*, **9**: 143–5. [PMID: 17199734]

Pickup JC, Sutton AJ (2008). Severe hypoglycaemia and glycaemic control in Type 1 diabetes: meta-analysis of multiple daily insulin injections compared with continuous subcutaneous insulin infusion. *Diabet Med*, **25**: 765–74. [PMID: 18644063]

Pullman J, Darsow T, Frias JP (2006). Pramlintide in the management of insulin-using patients with type 2 and type 1 diabetes. *Vasc Health Risk Manag*, **2**: 203–12. [PMID: 17326327]

Robertson EP, Sutherland DE, Lanz KJ (1999). Normoglycemia and preserved insulin secretory reserve in diabetic patients 10–18 years after pancreas transplantation. *Diabetes*, **48**: 1737–40. [PMID: 10480602]

Shapiro AM, Ricordi C, Hering BJ *et al.* (2006). International trial of the Edmonton protocol for islet transplantation. *N Engl J Med*, **355**: 1318–30. [PMID: 17005949]

Srinavasan P, Huang GC, Amiel SA, Heaton ND (2007). Islet cell transplantation. *Postgrad Med J*, **83**: 224–9. [PMID: 17403947]

Vella A, Rizza RA (2003). Metabolic disturbances in diabetes mellitus. Chapter 31 in: *Textbook of Diabetes*, 3rd edn. Pickup JC, Williams G (eds). Wiley-Blackwell. ISBN: 978-0-63-205915-7.

Further reading

American Diabetes Association (2004). Insulin administration. *Diabetes Care*, **27** (Suppl 1): S106–9. [PMID: 14693942]

American Diabetes Association (2004). Continuous subcutaneous insulin infusion. *Diabetes Care*, **27** (Suppl 1): S110. [PMID: 14693943]

Pickup JC (ed) (2009). *Insulin pump therapy and continuous glucose monitoring* (Oxford Diabetes Library), Oxford University Press. [ISBN: 978-0-63-205915-7]

Robertson P, Davis C, Larsen J, Stratta R, Sutherland DE; American Diabetes Association (2004). Pancreas transplantation in type 1 diabetes. *Diabetes Care*, **27** (Suppl 1): S105. [PMID: 14693941]

Robertson RP, Davis C, Larsen J, Stratta R, Sutherland DE; American Diabetes Association (2006). Pancreas and islet transplantation in type 1 diabetes. *Diabetes Care*, **29**: 935. [PMID: 16567844]

Chapter 5

Microvascular complications

> **Key points**
>
> - Hyperglycaemia damages the microvasculature through several mechanisms; strict control of hyperglycaemia remains overwhelmingly the most important factor in preventing and reversing microvascular complications in Type 1 diabetes.
> - End-stage microvascular complications (blindness, end-stage renal failure, amputations for neuropathic foot complications) are probably becoming less common; no single responsible factor can be identified.
> - The Diabetes Control and Complications Trial and the Epidemiology of Diabetes Interventions and Complications follow-up (1982–2006) confirmed dramatic and long-lasting benefits of intensive therapy on microvascular complications (40–60% risk reduction) with A1C consistently maintained at ~7% for ~7 yrs.

5.1 General mechanisms of microvascular complications

In Type 1 diabetes, hyperglycaemia is the only, or certainly the major factor causing microvascular damage. Glucose, a highly reactive molecule, appears to exert its toxic effects on the microvasculature through several mechanisms (Box 5.1 and Figure 5.1), though Brownlee and others have proposed that there may be a final common pathway for the different deleterious pathways via reactive oxygen species (ROS). The multiple candidate pathways explain the limited effectiveness of several classes of drugs designed to affect single mechanisms, and which in some cases, for example the aldose reductase inhibitors, have been in clinical trials for nearly 30 yrs. In addition, there may be some harmful products, for example advanced glycation end products (AGEs), which are generated so slowly that even if non-toxic drugs could be developed, they would need to be given for many years to demonstrate benefit. This view is supported by the fact that microvascular complications are very uncommon in the first

Box 5.1 Changing views of the mechanisms of microvascular damage in Type 1 diabetes (Brownlee 2005)

- *1960s*: the aldose reductase pathway. Intracellular aldose reductase, converting excess glucose to inactive alcohols (sorbitol and fructose), consumes NADPH, which reduces glutathione, an important antioxidant.
- *1970s*: AGEs. Glucose adducts to proteins with long half-lives, for example collagen, lipoproteins. These interact with cell surface AGE receptors, which then activate intracellular production of growth factors and cytokines. These are similar mechanisms to those exerted by:
- *1980s–1990s*: activation of β- and δ-isoforms of protein kinase C. These increase vasoactive substances, for example endothelin, VEGF, and pro-inflammatory genes via activation of NF (nuclear factor)-κB.
- *Late 1990s*: increased hexosamine pathway activity, leading to production of TGF-β1 and PAI-1, which impair rheology.
- Free fatty acids act via similar mechanisms (apart from the aldose reductase pathway) to generate ROS, stimulating the same adverse intracellular actions as for glucose; these may preferentially affect the macrovasculature.

Figure 5.1 Mechanisms of glucose-induced microvascular damage

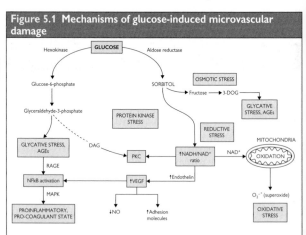

3-DOG, 3-Deoxyglucosone; DAG, Diacylglycerol; MAPK, MAP kinases; NO, Nitric oxide; PKC, Protein kinase C; RAGE, Receptor for AGE; VEGF, Vascular endothelial growth factor

even 10 yrs of Type 1 diabetes. This pessimistic therapeutic prospect is balanced by the evidence from the Diabetes Control and Complications Trial (DCCT)/Epidemiology of Diabetes Interventions and Complications (EDIC) of metabolic (glycaemic) memory in Type 1 diabetes, in which continuing microvascular benefits of antecedent periods of tight glycaemic control can be demonstrated for many years after glycaemia has been somewhat relaxed.

5.2 Blood glucose control

5.2.1 The Diabetes Control and Complications Trial (DCCT 1993)

A detailed understanding of this extraordinary and unique trial, the most far-reaching in the history of diabetes, is important for patients and professionals alike. Its primary aim was to examine in a long-term randomized controlled study whether intensive insulin treatment could reduce the risk of progression of microvascular complications over a long period (mean follow-up was 6.5 yr, range 4 to 9). It was conceived as long ago as 1975 (DCCT Research Group 1993), designed in 1982–1983, and after a feasibility phase, the full-scale trial started in 1985. The major microvascular outcomes were reported in 1993. The primary outcome studied was retinopathy, but nephropathy and neuropathy were also investigated in detail; there was a 40 to 60% risk reduction in all microvascular complications with intensive compared with conventional glycaemic control. Boxes 5.2 and 5.3 describe key clinical characteristics of the participants.

> **Box 5.2 Entry criteria and clinical characteristics of DCCT participants**
>
> - Total number of patients: 1441, recruited from 29 centres in USA and Canada
> - Age at entry: 13–39 yrs
> - *Intensively treated (n = 711)*—mean baseline A1C 9.1%, median achieved A1C 7.3% (mean blood glucose 8.6 mmol/L), mean total cholesterol 4.6 mmol/L, blood pressure (BP) 113/72
> - *Conventionally treated (n = 730)*—mean baseline A1C 9.1%, median achieved A1C 9.1% (mean blood glucose 12.8 mmol/L), mean total cholesterol 4.8 mmol/L, BP 115/73
> - *Primary prevention cohort (n = 726)*
>   - Duration <5 yrs, mean duration 2.5 yrs
>   - Absent retinopathy, albumin excretion rate (AER) <40 mg/24 h
> - *Secondary prevention cohort (n = 715)*
>   - Duration <15 yrs, mean duration 8.8 yrs; at least one retinal microaneurysm, AER <200 mg/24 h

5.2.2 DCCT stratification and implementation

The primary prevention cohort had no detectable retinopathy and AER <40 mg/24 h; the secondary prevention group had detectable background retinopathy and albuminuria <200 mg/24 h (these values therefore slightly differ from the conventional definitions of micro- and macroalbuminuria). Table 5.1 summarizes the main management features of both groups.

Table 5.1 Treatment strategies in the DCCT (DCCT Research Group 1995a)		
	Conventional	**Intensive**
Insulin regimen	Twice-daily free mixture	Treatment initiated as inpatient with CSII or MDI (≥3 daily injections with pen devices). Regimens changed as necessary
Frequency of follow-up	3 monthly	Weekly at first, then at least monthly; frequent telephone contact
Primary goals	Absence of symptoms of hyper- or hypoglycaemia, absent ketonuria, normal growth and development	Achieve and maintain as near non-diabetic glycaemic levels as possible and minimize hypoglycaemia
Glucose targets (Figure 5.2)	None set; investigator and patient masked to quarterly A1C; intervention only if >13%, or pregnancy/pregnancy planned Initially urine testing From 1986: ≥1 self-monitoring of blood glucose (SMBG) test daily	≥4 times daily SMBG (three preprandial, one bedtime) Weekly 3.00 a.m. measurement BG targets: • Fasting/preprandial: 3.9–6.7 mmol/L • Postprandial (90–120 min after meal) <10 mmol/L • 3.00 a.m.: >3.6 mmol/L • A1C target: <6.05 (within 2SD of non-diabetic mean)
Diet	Meal plans prescribed by dietitian; diet composition goals established. Step 1 NCEP diet from 1988	Conventional dietetic input, with additional emphasis on carbohydrate (CHO) exchanges, CHO counting, healthy eating choices, and problem-solving approach to food, activity, and insulin. Aim: to adjust insulin doses in response to these factors
Exercise	Encouraged, general education on insulin dose adjustment, and avoiding hypoglycaemia	Encouraged: no specific exercise plan. Specific education on adjustment to MDI and CSII to maintain glycaemic goals and avoid hypoglycaemia

5.2.3 Epidemiology of Diabetes Interventions and Complications (EDIC 1994–2006)

After DCCT close-out, the EDIC study, possibly even more informative, followed up the great majority of DCCT participants, under non-randomized conditions with all participants being encouraged to adopt intensive management (mean achieved A1C 8.1% to 8.2% in both groups). Microvascular complications continued to be studied in detail, but critical information on the progression of macrovascular disease is the major notable outcome (see Chapter 6), especially as there were few interventions other than glycaemic control (Figure 5.2).

5.2.4 Glycaemic threshold

An intense debate in the early 1990s centred around the question of whether there was a glycaemic threshold for the development of microvascular complications in Type 1 diabetes. A retrospective analysis suggested that there was little appreciable decreased risk of developing retinopathy and microalbuminuria with A1C levels lower than ~8%. However, a comprehensive analysis of the DCCT confirmed:

- A strict log–linear (exponential) relationship between A1C and both retinopathy and microalbuminuria. For retinopathy this represented a consistent 39% risk reduction for each 10% reduction in A1C
- Absolute risk reduction was greater when high A1C values are reduced
- There is no evidence for a glycaemic threshold, and this is supported by other studies, for example WESDR, Stockholm Intervention Study, Berlin Retinopathy Study. However, some have suggested a threshold for the development of proliferative retinopathy. Though there were insufficient cases in DCCT to confirm this, there was no demonstrable threshold for the development of severe non-proliferative retinopathy (DCCT Research Group 1996).

71

Box 5.3 Other characteristics of the DCCT cohort

- Smokers: 18%
- Adolescents (age 13–17 yrs): 13% (*n* = 195)
- Mean IQ: 113; 73% had some post-secondary schooling
- Married: 50%
- Pregnancies: 270 in 150 women, mean age at pregnancy 23–25 yrs
- CSII used by 30%–42% of intensive group in any year
- Median calorie intake: 1900–2100 (intensive), 1900–2300 (conventional)

Figure 5.2 (a) A1C and (b) SMBG in the intensive and conventional control groups during DCCT and (c) A1C at DCCT close-out and during years 1–4 of EDIC

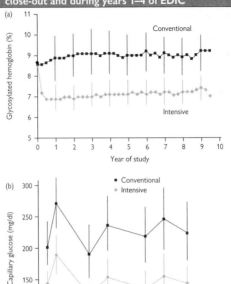

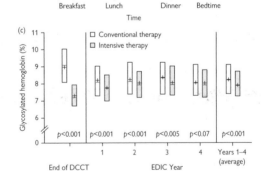

(a) The rigorously maintained difference in A1C of ~2% throughout the DCCT has more recently become the paradigm for glycaemic control studies in Type 2 diabetes. (b) 7-point SMBG showing postprandial excursions, characteristically greatest after breakfast during DCCT. (c) A1C during years 1-4 of EDIC after DCCT close-out, showing the rapid reduction in difference between the two groups, converging at ~8%, and becoming non-statistically significant by year 4. (a,b) The DCCT Research Group (1993). Copyright © 1993 Massachusetts Medical Society. All rights reserved. (c) The DCCT/EDIC Research Group (2000). Copyright © 2000 Massachusetts Medical Society. All rights reserved.

5.2.5 β-**Cell function and diabetes-related complications**

About 60% of DCCT participants had a short duration of diabetes (1 to 5 yrs) at baseline, and 35% of these had a detectable C-peptide response to a mixed meal. The investigators estimated that instituting intensive therapy in this group with preserved (but not high) C-peptide levels prolonged β-cell function for two or more years, though it was lost completely even in these patients by study years 5 to 6. Intensively treated patients with preserved C-peptide responses had a lower A1C than non-responders, and this fully explained their substantially lower risk of development and progression of both retinopathy and microalbuminuria. In addition, they had a much lower risk of severe hypoglycaemia than non-responders (DCCT Research Group 1998). There has been much interest in whether C-peptide itself may be bioactive in preventing microvascular complications (small studies using recombinant C-peptide have shown improvement in nerve conduction measurements and also in early diabetic nephropathy). This was not thought to be an operative factor in the DCCT, but the message remains that intensive treatment as soon as possible after diagnosis carries long-term microvascular advantage. Since potential DCCT participants with well-preserved C-peptide responses were excluded from the main study, these results may underestimate the benefits of early intensive treatment in the routine clinical setting. Pre- and postpubertal duration of glycaemia and their role in microvascular complications are considered in more detail in Chapter 7.

5.3 **Retinopathy**

5.3.1 **Epidemiology**

Retinopathy, like nephropathy, proceeds differently in Type 1 compared with Type 2 diabetes. In the relatively old Wisconsin study (1984), proliferative retinopathy was not seen with less than 5 yrs duration, and more recent studies do not describe proliferative changes within the first 10 yrs (e.g. Skrivarhaug *et al.* 2006). This translates into the ADA Position Statement on retinopathy screening—the first dilated eye examination is not needed until 3 to 5 yrs after diagnosis. However, in patients with duration less than 5 yrs screened for the DCCT, two-thirds had some evidence of retinopathy. Fluorescein angiography identified retinopathy in ~20% of patients who had no photographic evidence of retinopathy (Malone *et al.* 2001), and there was a very small number (~0.4%) with pre-proliferative or worse retinopathy. Patients with adult-onset Type 1 diabetes should therefore have annual retinopathy screening from diagnosis, though the likelihood of uncovering sight-threatening retinopathy is extremely low.

In the Wisconsin study the cumulative prevalence of retinopathy of any degree increased rapidly with increasing diabetes duration, reaching nearly 100% by 15 yrs (Klein *et al.* 1984); proliferative retinopathy rose rapidly between 10 and 25 yrs duration, peaking at about 60% between 20 and 35 yrs duration. Much lower prevalences are now seen, and it is clear that the natural history of retinopathy is changing, especially in childhood onset diabetes:

- The cumulative incidence of proliferative retinopathy after 25 yrs follow-up in the Oslo study (final examination in 2002–2003) was only 11%, though nearly all patients (90%) had some retinopathy (Skrivarhaug *et al.* 2006).
- Three cross-sectional cohort studies in adolescents in Sydney studied between 1990 and 2002 showed a reduction of about 50% in the prevalence of early retinopathy—though, intriguingly, median A1C was unchanged (8.4% to 8.5%) (Mohsin *et al.* 2005; see Chapter 7)
- The Linköping Study (Sweden) showed a similar progressive reduction in cumulative laser-treated retinopathy rates 25 yrs after childhood diagnosis—47% in the cohort diagnosed in 1961–1965, 24% in those diagnosed in 1971–1975 (Nordwall *et al.* 2004).

Indicators of insulin resistance are associated with diabetic retinopathy in follow-up studies, for example waist–hip ratio and triglycerides in EURODIAB (Chaturvedi *et al.* 2001), and this is a consistent feature of studies of microvascular complications and neuropathy. Interestingly, standard cardiovascular risk factors (BP, the presence of cardiovascular disease, or smoking) did not seem to be associated with progression to retinopathy in the same study.

5.3.2 **Non-proliferative diabetic retinopathy (NPDR)**

5.3.2.1 *Mild NPDR*

Red lesions—dot and blot haemorrhages—are the characteristic early lesions of Type 1 diabetes. Dot haemorrhages (microaneurysms) are seen most frequently at the posterior pole of the eye. Red lesions are prognostic—the greater the number, the higher the risk of eventually requiring laser treatment. Clinically, flitting microaneurysms are quite common in Type 1 diabetes—this may reflect disturbed retinal haemodynamics related to glycaemic variation, and even the larger blot and flame-shaped haemorrhages, especially those around the disc, can regress spontaneously with no apparent improvement in glycaemic control.

5.3.2.2 *Severe NPDR—the 4:2:1 rule*

Any of the following, in the absence of proliferative changes:

- >20 intraretinal blot haemorrhages in each of 4 quadrants
- Definite venous beading in 2 or more quadrants
- Prominent intraretinal microvascular abnormalities (IRMA) in 1 or more quadrant. Difficult to spot by the non-specialist, they are abnormal vessels resembling new vessels, but are intraretinal and do not lead to preretinal or vitreous haemorrhage.

5.3.2.3 *Management of NPDR*

There is no visual impairment, and although moderate or severe NPDR requires close ophthalmological follow-up, any degree of persistent retinopathy indicates suboptimal glycaemic control and a high risk of other microvascular complications. For example, the DCCT estimated that the cumulative 9-yr risk of retinopathy progression was 20% at a constant A1C level of 8%, 11% at 7%, but only 5.5% at 6% (DCCT Research Group 1996). Other than strict glycaemic control, there is no clear evidence for additional, non-insulin treatment in mild NPDR, though the 2-yr EUCLID study within EURODIAB (1998) hinted that angiotensin converting enzyme inhibitor (ACEi) treatment with lisinopril was associated with a reduced risk of incidence and progression of retinopathy.

EUCLID's findings were partly reinforced by the results of DIabetic Retinopathy Candesartan Trials (DIRECT)-Prevent 1 (2008), a formal primary prevention study in patients with mean duration 6.5 yrs, age 30 yrs, and A1C 8.1%, who had no baseline retinopathy or microalbuminuria. It demonstrated a modest but just statistically significant 12% adjusted risk reduction in the incidence of two-step ETDRS retinopathy change with the angiotensin receptor blocking (ARB) agent candesartan 32 mg daily. Four to five years of treatment were required to demonstrate the effect, which was independent of the substantial BP lowering seen (~3/3 mm Hg) in this strictly normotensive group (mean BP 116/72). Both losartan 100 mg and enalapril 20 mg daily given for the same length of time (5 yr) also reduced the progression of retinopathy in a much smaller study, nevertheless hinting at a broader potential for angiotensin blockade in both primary and secondary prevention of retinopathy, though increased numbers of RCTs do not seem to be aiding clinical decisions in this important area (Mauer *et al* 2009). There was no benefit on progression or regression in a secondary prevention cohort with established mild-to-moderate NPDR (DIRECT-Protect 1), mean A1C slightly higher than in DIRECT-Prevent 1 (8.5%), although in both studies there was globally a significant improvement in ETDRS score. Primary candesartan treatment in Type 1 patients in poor glycaemic control may reduce the risk of developing retinopathy (Wright and Dodson 2010), but the benefit is limited, may be long-delayed, and the DCCT results suggest that a ~1% improvement in A1C sustained over a similar period would be quantitatively more beneficial. Once retinopathy has developed, DIRECT confirms that glycaemic improvement is the only means of preventing progression (Chaturvedi *et al.* 2008). There is no evidence for the routine use of aspirin, antihypertensives, or statins in retinopathy beyond their standard indications.

5.3.3 **Pre-proliferative retinopathy**

Features carrying an increased risk of proliferation, or with a significant risk of developing sight-threatening retinopathy within a year include:

- Venous beading, looping, or reduplication
- Multiple (>5) cotton wool spots
- Multiple haemorrhages
- IRMAs.

This level of retinopathy is not frequently encountered in Type 1 patients in western practice, and should prompt a detailed evaluation for other microvascular complications—and macrovascular complications in these patients who are likely to have at least 10 to 15 yrs of diabetes duration in poor or very poor glycaemic control.

5.3.3.1 *Treatment*

Panretinal (scatter) laser photocoagulation at this stage reduces the risk of severe visual loss by about 50%. It is presumed, but not known, that improved glycaemic control at this stage will improve visual outcomes (though there is a risk of transient further deterioration—see below). Hypertension, which may not be overt, should be actively sought, preferably with the use of ambulatory BP monitoring (ABPM) and centile BP measurements in children and adolescents.

5.3.4 **Proliferative retinopathy and its complications**

Retinal neovascularization, the hallmark advanced retinal lesion of Type 1 diabetes, arises from retinal veins, usually at a bifurcation. Disc neovascularization (NVD) carries a worse visual prognosis than new vessels elsewhere (NVE). Growth factors, especially vascular endothelial growth factor (VEGF), released from the ischaemic retina lead to proliferation of vessels, which lie in the preretinal space, between the retina and the posterior surface of the vitreous gel. They may bleed into the preretinal space, causing characteristic boat-shaped (fluid level) haemorrhages, or into the vitreous, resulting in large amorphous haemorrhages often causing severe acute visual loss. Panretinal photocoagulation is standard treatment. Trials of intravitreal anti-VEGF agents (e.g. pegaptanib, ranibizumab, and bevacizumab) are underway, though they are currently used off-license.

5.3.5 **Maculopathy**

Although considered characteristic of retinopathy in Type 2 diabetes, maculopathy is not uncommon in Type 1 diabetes. In one study, focal macular oedema was found cumulatively in 12% of patients followed up for 15 yrs, and diffuse macular oedema in 9%. In addition to poor glycaemic control, elevated low-density lipoprotein (LDL), hypertension, and proteinuria are associated with this complication—similar to the risk factors in Type 2 diabetes. On ophthalmoscopy or retinal photography maculopathy can be inferred from the presence of circinate exudates, but macular oedema requires slit-lamp examination or optical coherence tomography (OCT) for accurate determination, and assessment of macular ischaemia requires fluorescein angiography. All vascular risk factors must be addressed, but there is no good evidence that this improves the visual outcome. Intravitreal steroids may be of benefit, and are widely used. The protein kinase C β-inhibitor ruboxistaurin reduces the risk of visual loss in macular oedema, but the future of this compound is currently uncertain.

5.3.6 Advanced diabetic eye disease and visual loss

Fear of visual loss is common, recurrent, and pervasive in many people with diabetes, and is largely independent of objective measures of visual acuity and retinopathy. The fear is rarely articulated spontaneously, and must be recognized by the diabetes team. Visual loss caused by advanced diabetic eye disease in Type 1 diabetes is usually due to complications of proliferative retinopathy, caused by a fibrovascular response to retinal ischaemia and preretinal haemorrhage, but early intervention with increasingly sophisticated vitreo-retinal surgical techniques has improved the visual prognosis. Rubeotic glaucoma secondary to iris neovascularization is fortunately now extremely rare. The EURODIAB study, reporting in the mid-1990s, found that severe visual impairment (visual acuity 6/60 or less in the better eye) was present in 2.3% of patients. A similar proportion of younger onset (mostly Type 1) patients with blindness (2.4%) was found in the older Wisconsin study. Retinal screening programmes can potentially virtually eliminate severe visual loss due to diabetic retinopathy in Type 1 diabetes.

5.3.7 Effect of rapid glycaemic improvement on retinopathy

After rapid improvement in glycaemic control, initial deterioration in retinopathy, even to the point of proliferation, is well recognized, and was first described in early studies (e.g. Steno 1983; Kroc 1984, where patients already had established background retinopathy). The Oslo group (1985) found that development of the characteristic cotton wool spots was more frequent in women with A1 falls of ~3%. Lesions developed in the first 3 to 6 months, and in most cases had resolved by 12 months. All studies have shown eventual regression of lesions, with improved retinal outcome through better glycaemic control. In the DCCT, 'early worsening' (three or more ETDRS steps in the first 12 months) occurred in 13% of intensively treated patients, and 8% of conventionally treated patients, though there was no serious visual loss, despite three cases of proliferative retinopathy and two of clinically significant macular oedema. Nevertheless, whenever intensive treatment starts, particularly in those with very poor baseline glycaemia, regardless of the degree of baseline retinopathy—the secondary prevention DCCT group had relatively minor retinopathy—close retinal monitoring is important. The DCCT group suggests three-monthly monitoring in high-risk groups, such as:

• In the preconception period and early pregnancy
• Patients starting CSII or any intensified insulin therapy when in poor control
• Any patient with known retinopathy where there has been a rapid and substantial fall in A1C (e.g. >2%)—for whatever reason.

5.4 Diabetic renal disease

5.4.1 Natural history

There is an extensive literature on the epidemiology and natural history of renal disease in Type 1 diabetes, though in comparison with Type 2 diabetes, relatively little randomized controlled trial (RCT) evidence. Once macroalbuminuria is established, clinically there is little to distinguish between Type 1 and Type 2 diabetes, but they are very different conditions at earlier stages.

In most studies, the peak incidence of diabetic nephropathy in Type 1 patients occurs 25 to 30 yrs after diagnosis. Recent data indicate that end-stage renal disease (ESRD), at least in advanced Western countries, is now uncommon, for example fewer than 1% of Swedish patients diagnosed with diabetes between 1977 and 1985. The generally encouraging trend is confirmed by the stable rates for dialysis take-on in Type 1 patients across Europe during the 1990s, despite rising prevalence and longer overall survival rates. This is in striking contrast with Type 2 diabetes. Although the data for diabetic nephropathy, as opposed to ESRD, are less consistent, the Steno centre has documented a progressive decrease of more than 50% in cohorts with 20 yrs of diabetes diagnosed over a relatively short period, from the mid-1960s to the late 1970s (Rossing 2005), and practically identical results have emerged in the Linköping study from Sweden. It is widely thought that progression from nephropathy to ESRD is being at least delayed, if not prevented, probably through a combination of improved glycaemic and BP control, and declining rates of smoking.

5.4.1.1 Early

A non-diabetic renal diagnosis should be pursued in any patient with proteinuria within the first 5 yrs of Type 1 diabetes (there are no specific associated autoimmune renal diseases, though there is a hint that IgA nephropathy may be more frequent). However, the absence of significant proteinuria in the early stages is confirmed in the DCCT, where the primary prevention cohort (mean duration 2.5 yrs) had a mean AER of 12 mg/24 h, while the secondary prevention cohort (mean duration 9 yrs) had a mean AER ~20 mg/24 h—both groups below the DCCT definition of microalbuminuria (<40 mg/24 h; see below). By DCCT close-out, at a mean duration of 12 yrs, >90% of the intensively treated group were normoalbuminuric, compared with ~85% of the conventionally treated group. While AER is low up to 10 yrs after diagnosis, abnormal renal morphology on biopsy is evident in young people, and is associated with lack of nocturnal dipping in ambulatory BP studies. Moreover, there are well-documented functional renal changes even shortly after diagnosis, including renal hypertrophy and hyperfiltration, indicated by elevated glomerular filteration rate (eGFR) (>135 to 150 mL/min). Hypertrophy may precede hyperfiltration, but when they occur together, they are associated with increased risk of progression to nephropathy; they may in future be more reliable indicators of risk than microalbuminuria, which has a high rate of spontaneous regression (see below; Zerbini et al. 2006).

Concern about the arbitrary range used for the definition of microalbuminuria with respect to renal and cardiovascular outcomes largely derives from studies in Type 2 diabetes, where there is strong evidence that low-level AER, even below the detection limits of current assays, may be associated with increased cardiovascular risk. Likewise, across the tenfold range of AER that constitutes microalbuminuria (30 to 300 mg/24 h) there is likely to be a marked increased risk of both ESRD and cardiovascular events, and some use AER ~100 mg/24 h as an indicator of 'mid-range' microalbuminuria that should be regarded as high risk (Box 5.4).

5.4.1.2 Microalbuminuria: progression, regression, and the role of ACEi and ARB treatment

Early studies in the 1980s suggested that microalbuminuria led to overt proteinuria in most patients, between 60% and 85%, after 6 to 14 yrs duration. Guidelines from the early 1990s therefore urged ACEi treatment for all microalbuminuric Type 1 patients (~60% risk reduction in progression to proteinuria, and a threefold increased rate of regression to normoalbuminuria: The ACE Inhibitors in Diabetic Nephropathy Trialist Group 2001). In the ATLANTIS study (2000) Type 1 patients with mid-range microalbuminuria (50 to 60 µg/min, ~75 to 90 mg/24 h) more frequently regressed to normoalbuminuria after 2 yrs of low-dose ramipril, 1.25 or 5 mg daily.

More recently, this simple view—high rates of microalbuminuria developing in the second decade of Type 1 diabetes, progressing with high likelihood to overt nephropathy, and a substantial reduction in this risk with angiotensin blockade treatment—has been complicated by several studies that paint a more variable picture of the natural history of microalbuminuria. Regression independent of ACEi treatment has been demonstrated, even in some cases of heavy proteinuria, in ~60% of patients after 6 yrs follow-up (Perkins et al. 2003). Regression was associated with lower systolic BP, and lower A1C, triglycerides, and total cholesterol—but this was an observational

Box 5.4 Urinary albumin excretion—definitions and methods

Definitions:

- *Normoalbuminuria*: normal range usually quoted as 1.5–20 µg/min (geometric mean 6.5 µg/min, ≈10 mg/24 h is around the detection limit of most assays, though very low-level microalbuminuria may be of significance)
- *Microalbuminuria*
  - (a) 30–299 mg/24 h (DCCT: >40 mg/24 h)
  - (b) 20–199 µg/min
  - (c) Albumin:creatinine ratio (ACR) 2.5–30 (male), 3.5–30 (female) mg/mmol (≥22.1 mg/g (male), ≥30.9 mg/g (female); to convert from SI to conventional units multiply by 8.8. There may be intermittent stick-positive proteinuria
- *Macroalbuminuria*
  - (a) ≥300 mg/24 h
  - (b) ≥200 µg/min
  - (c) ACR >30 mg/mmol
  - (d) Urinary *protein* excretion >500 mg/24 h (urinary albumin ~70% of total urinary protein). There is invariable stick-positive proteinuria
- *Nephrotic-range proteinuria*: >3.5g/24 h (2.2g albumin/24 h; ACR >2.2g/g)

Methods:

- 24-h urinary albumin excretion (mg/24 h)
- Timed (usually overnight) collection—less used these days (µg/min)
- Spot early morning urine specimen for ACR—albumin excretion corrected for urine flow

study, not an RCT. On the other hand, even after 30 yrs of uncomplicated Type 1 diabetes, around one quarter of patients developed new microalbuminuria or proteinuria over a further 7 yr follow-up, so continuing careful follow-up is required in all patients. An 11 yr prospective audit from Steno (Schjoedt *et al.* 2008) of patients with a mean baseline AER of 65 mg/24 h, and treated intensively with angiotensin blocking agents or strict control of hypertension with other agents, found a very low annual rate, 1.7%, progressing from micro- to macroalbuminuria, while more than half remained microalbuminuric, and nearly a third regressed to normoalbuminuria. Finally, although unusual, some patients may progress to moderate renal impairment without proteinuria (Costacou *et al.* 2007).

Accordingly, it is difficult to specify strict protocols for management of microalbuminuria in Type 1 patients, especially where there are no other complications (Box 5.5). The variability of all methods

> **Box 5.5 Approach to microalbuminuria in Type 1 diabetes**
>
> - Annual screening from diagnosis, using early morning ACR
> - If >30 (macroalbuminuria): confirm with repeat or 24-h urinary albumin
> - If 2.5/3.5–30, confirm microalbuminuria: ensure stable A1C, exclude urinary tract or systemic infection, recent DKA, etc., and repeat ACR twice over 6–12 weeks
> - If >2 positive, then microalbuminuria confirmed
> - If high-grade (e.g. ACR >10) → ACEi to maximum recommended dose
> - If lower grade microalbuminuria and strictly normotensive (<120/80) ensure optimum glycaemia, non-smoking status, and review frequently. Statins and aspirin are usually recommended
> - Further stratification may be achieved using 24-h ambulatory BP testing: if normal, with adequate nocturnal dip, then careful observation, looking to possibility of regression, is justified
> - In contrast with Type 2 diabetes, there is no RCT evidence for 'renoprotection' with ACEi or ARB treatment in strictly normotensive non-microalbuminuric Type 1 patients (DIRECT-Renal 2008, Mauer et al. 2009)

for measuring AER must be recognized—between 10% and 60%—and a balanced decision arrived at on the basis of sufficient numbers of samples and the individual clinical circumstances. The primary therapeutic approach should be glycaemic control, not angiotensin blockade treatment, especially in lower-grade microalbuminuria: DCCT and other studies confirm that glycaemia is the major, possibly the sole, determinant of progression to microalbuminuria. There is no primary prevention role for angiotensin blockade treatment in normotensive, non-microalbuminuric Type 1 patients: candesartan 32 mg daily given for 4 yrs in the DIRECT-Renal study (2008) of both Type 1 and Type 2 patients did not reduce the risk of progression to microalbuminuria in patients with near-undetectable albuminuria (median AER 5 μg/min (~7.5 mg/24 h), and neither losartan 100 mg nor enalapril 20 mg daily for 5 yr had any effect in preventing microalbuminuria in normotensive patients without hypertension (Mauer et al. 2009). Even where has not been a significant change in A1C with time, there appears to be a continuing and gratifying, if unexplained, decline in recent years in the prevalence of both early retinopathy and low-level microalbuminuria (Mohsin et al. 2005). However, there is no room for complacency: a study in Oxford, for example, found microalbuminuria in 34% of adult onset patients after a mean follow-up of 18 yrs, and an even higher rate (50%) in those with childhood onset diabetes after a shorter mean follow-up of 10 yrs, reflecting consistently poor glycae-mic control (mean A1C 9.7% to 11.5%; Amin *et al.* 2008).

5.4.1.3 *Late—macroalbuminuria/proteinuria/nephropathy*

By the end of DCCT, though microalbuminuria was more frequent in the conventional compared with the intensive group (13% vs 8%), the prevalence of macroalbuminuria was very low, and not significantly different between the two groups (conventional 3%, intensive 1.5%). However, the separation between the two groups progressed so that at EDIC years 7 to 8, microalbuminuria prevalence was ~23% vs 11%, clinical albuminuria 9.4% vs 1.4% (risk reduction 84%). Never-theless, even with this duration of follow-up, dialysis and transplanta-tion were very infrequent (cumulative prevalence 0.3% to 1.6%). There was no difference in the use of ACEi treatment either at the start of EDIC (conventional 7%, intensive 6%), or the end (con-ventional 29%, intensive 22%), confirming the primacy of glycaemic control in preventing progression of micro- to macroalbuminuria.

5.4.1.4 *Progression and remission of nephropathy*

Once nephropathy is established, GFR falls 10 to 12 mL/min/yr (compare ~1 mL/min/yr in non-diabetic individuals). ACEi treatment was first shown to be of benefit in 1993 in reducing renal and cardio-vascular endpoints and death in patients with established diabetic nephropathy (serum creatinine >130 µmol/L, proteinuria ~2 g/day), despite similar BP in the control group. Benefit was greater in those with impaired renal function, but no different in hypertensive and non-hypertensive subjects (Lewis *et al.* 1993). Large recent studies in Type 2 diabetes have shown an increased risk of rapid progression of renal impairment with albuminuria exceeding 1 g/24 h. Conversely, it is important to recognize the very small proportion of patients (1% to 2% in DCCT/EDIC) with impaired renal function (eGFR <60 mL/min) who remain persistently negative for microalbuminuria over a long period. There are no clear phenotypic differences from microalbu-minuric or proteinuric patients, and the cause of the renal impairment is not known. There will be small numbers of patients without mi-croalbuminuria who will have remitted either spontaneously or after prolonged angiotensin blockade treatment, but who will have had proteinuria in the distant past. Broad management strategies for nephropathy are outlined in Box 5.6.

Remission (persistent decrease in albuminuria, often defined as <600 mg/24 h) and regression (fall in GFR to no greater than seen in normal aging) occur in about 20% to 30% of patients when BP is reduced to 135/80 or lower; normotensive patients with 0.8 to 1 g proteinuria also benefit from ACEi treatment with low rates of decrease in GFR, so long as BP is maintained at ~130/75. About 20% of patients with nephrotic-range proteinuria can be brought into remission with persistent ACEi treatment.

Box 5.6 **Management of nephropathy in Type 1 patients**

- *Maximum ACEi treatment*: consider combined ACEi/ARB in heavy proteinuria/nephrotic syndrome (?combined ARB/aliskiren in patients with ACEi side effects), possibly aldosterone antagonist
- *Rigorous BP control*: e.g. <125/75; frequent ambulatory BP studies
- *Optimize glycaemic control*
- *Manage all cardiovascular risk factors*: LDL target <1.7; aspirin; proactively investigate for ischaemic heart disease; emphasize smoking cessation
- *Reduce protein intake*—difficult in clinical practice, but the advice is to reduce protein intake to ~0.8 to 1.0 g/kg body weight/day, emphasizing vegetable protein
- *Refer to specialist renal clinic* when serum creatinine ~150 µmol/L, or eGFR ~40–50 mL/min, with particular emphasis on management of anaemia and renal bone disease (check ferritin, bone screen, PTH, vitamin B12, folate). Ensure iron repletion (intravenous iron is often valuable) before considering erythropoeitin-stimulating agents. Current evidence, at least in Type 2 diabetes, is to correct haemoglobin to ~11 g/dL, and not higher (TREAT, 2009). Joint diabetes-renal clinics may be valuable

5.4.1.5 *Angiotensin blockade and other antiproteinuric agents*

Although ARBs are likely to be as effective as ACEi in reducing proteinuria in Type 1 patients (their equivalence has been demonstrated in Type 2), ACEi inhibitors should always be first-line treatment, moving to an ARB only if there is ACEi-induced cough (ACE-induced angio-oedema is a contra-indication to ARBs). Early studies used captopril and enalapril, and while effective, they require more than once-daily dosing. Lisinopril (up to 20 to 40 mg daily), perindopril (up to 8 mg daily), and ramipril (up to 10 mg daily) are suitable for once-daily treatment. As well as their renal benefit, both ACEi and ARBs are associated with a lower risk of progression of coronary artery calcification in albuminuric Type 1 patients, an effect probably independent of BP reduction. Beta blockers and thiazide diuretics, and in most studies in Type 2 patients, non-dihydropyridine calcium channel blockers (diltiazem and verapamil), but not dihydropyridines, reduce proteinuria. However, in one study amlodipine or candesartan added to maximum ACEi both significantly further reduced proteinuria in Type 1 patients. Combined treatment with ACEi and ARB in proteinuric patients has been widely used, but there is no RCT evidence for its benefit beyond intermediate measures of proteinuria reduction. ONTARGET (2008), which used ramipril and telmisartan, admittedly in non-diabetic patients without heavy proteinuria, nevertheless increased the risk of hard renal endpoints, including death. Dual angiotensin blockade (and ARB combined with the direct renin inhibitor aliskiren) requires specialist initiation and follow up. Low-dose spironolactone, 25 mg daily, reduces proteinuria—but also has some antihypertensive effect—in patients with nephropathy already taking maximum angiotensin blockade, but it is not licensed for this indication, and must be used with great care; it is anti-androgenic, men frequently get painful gynaecomastia even with low doses, it cannot be used in women of child-bearing age without reliable contraception, and serum potassium, already often elevated (e.g. 5.3 to 5.5 mmol/L) in these patients with hyporeninaemic hypoaldosteronism (type 4 renal tubular acidosis), must be monitored frequently.

5.4.1.6 *Renal replacement therapy*

Continuous ambulatory peritoneal dialysis (CAPD) is preferred in diabetic patients, as it seems to carry a better prognosis for survival. However, increasing concern about the serious side effect of sclerosing peritonitis has damped enthusiasm for CAPD, despite the difficulties of vascular access for haemodialysis because of calcification of distal vessels. Advanced retinopathy is frequent in dialysis patients, as is ischaemic heart disease (often asymptomatic), heart failure, left ventricular hypertrophy, and peripheral vascular disease (PVD); all require active management. Cadaveric renal transplantation is routine; live-related donation is highly successful and becoming more common, as are combined renal-pancreas transplants (see Section 4.8.2).

5.5 Neuropathy

While the general mechanisms of microvascular complications also apply to neuropathy, it is generally regarded as a separate complication, even though there is good evidence that endoneurial hypoxia secondary to microangiopathy is an important component of the pathogenesis. The three non-macrovascular complications tend to proceed together, but diagnostic methods are different. In neuropathy, quantitative methods are more complex, and much less used routinely, compared with retinopathy and nephropathy. Neuropathy, therefore, is less frequently diagnosed until there are advanced clinical manifestations. Neuropathic syndromes, both somatic sensorimotor and autonomic, are similar to those in Type 2 diabetes, but as with all aspects of Type 1 diabetes, certain manifestations seem to be characteristic (e.g. cranial mononeuropathies, gastroenteropathy, Charcot neuroarthropathy), and may be related to subtly different neuropathology in Type 1 diabetes.

5.5.1 **Pathophysiology**

It is generally thought that a reversible 'metabolic' phase of peripheral neuropathy is soon followed by structural changes resulting in predominantly distal fibre loss. Axonal loss is early and more severe; demyelination, the process detected by routine nerve conduction studies, occurs later. Cutaneous nerve-fibre depletion—distal small fibre loss—occurs in short-duration Type 1 diabetes. However, central processes are also involved; spinal cord atrophy, with decreased cross-sectional spinal cord areas, has been demontrated on magnetic resonance imaging (MRI).

5.5.2 **Epidemiology and natural history**

The natural history of neuropathy is difficult to reliably document because of the methodological difficulties. In most studies, standardized symptom questionnaires and examinations, and neurophysiological, sensory, and autonomic testing, or a combination of these, are usually used. Prevalence data therefore vary widely, and the natural history appears to be changing much as it is in other microvascular complications, with older studies probably overestimating current prevalence. However, even in a contemporary adolescent population, the prevalence of electrophysiological and autonomic abnormalities is between 20% and 25%.

5.5.2.1 *Neuropathy in DCCT*

The detailed baseline examinations detected definite clinical neuroathy in 5% to 6% of the primary prevention cohort, and 13% of the secondary prevention cohort (The DCCT Research Group 1995b), though the prevalence was much lower if there were both clinical and neurophysiological/autonomic abnormalities. At DCCT close-out 15% of the intensive, and 23% of the conventional group, had definite clinical neuropathy (Martin *et al.* 2006). In EDIC, only a standardized questionnaire and clinical examination was used, so results are not comparable with DCCT, but symptoms (questionnaire positivity) continued to increase steadily in both groups for the next 8 yrs (at a greater rate in the conventional group), while clinical signs (examination) remained unchanged over the same period.

5.5.3 **Diagnosis**

5.5.3.1 *Symptoms and signs*

Typical neuropathic symptoms are elicited by the simple questions contained in the Michigan Neuropathy Screening Instrument (MNSI), for example:

* *Negative symptoms*: numbness, temperature discrimination (water), weakness
* *Positive symptoms*: burning pain, hyperaesthesiae, paraesthesia, worsening of symptoms at night
* *Medical diagnosis* of neuropathy, previous amputation or ulcer.

A questionnaire score >2 indicates neuropathy. The Michigan Diabetic Neuropathy Score (MDNS) includes a clinical examination (foot abnormalities, vibration perception with a tuning fork, monofilament testing, and ankle reflexes) and neurophysiological examination. The DCCT used the MNSI only (Feldman *et al.* 1994).

5.5.3.2 *Quantitative and semi-quantitative measurements*

• *10 g Semmes-Weinstein monofilament*: the filament is applied to bending point, perpendicularly and briefly to the skin of the dorsum of the great toe between nail fold and the distal interpalangeal joint. Eight or more correct responses out of ten is considered normal; 1 to 7 indicates reduced sensation, 0 absent sensation. Decreased monofilament sensation is associated with increased risk of foot ulceration

• *Neurothesiometer* (Figures 5.3 and 5.4): the simplest and most reliable quantitative sensory test—a quantitative vibration perception threshold. Measurements correlate fairly well with all other measurements, including nerve conduction studies and other sensory thresholds (e.g. thermal). Inability to feel an applied voltage of 25 implies severe neuropathy and risk of neuropathic ulceration. Age-related ranges should be used, especially in younger Type 1 patients, or significant neuropathy may be missed (Bloom *et al.* 1984)

• *Nerve conduction studies*: too complex and time-consuming for routine use, but if requested for another reason, for example, diagnosis of carpal tunnel syndrome (CTS), request lower limb sural sensory and peroneal motor nerve studies for documentary purposes

• *Autonomic function testing*: again, too complex for routine use, but helpful to confirm a diagnosis of autonomic neuropathy in patients presenting for example with symptoms of gastroparesis. The overall prevalence of abnormal autonomic function tests is high, around 20%. Tests involving measurement of heart rate changes reflect vagal involvement, while BP tests reflect sympathetic abnormalities—usually present only in advanced neuropathy. The simplest vagal test is heart rate variation (sinus arrhythmia) in response to standardized deep breathing (5 s inspiration, 5 s expiration). Systolic BP fall after standing will detect orthostatic hypotension. Simplified normal ranges (after Ewing and Clarke) are shown in Table 5.2. Abnormal autonomic function has clear prognostic implications; for example, abnormal heart rate variation to deep breathing is associated with increased risks of both myocardial infarction and mortality.

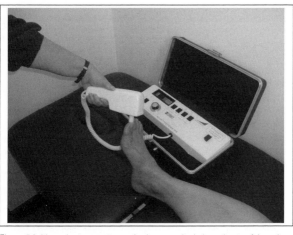

Figure 5.3 Neurothesiometer in use. Apply perpendicularly to the tip of the pulp of the great toe, without contacting the nail, having tested the sensation at the sternum. Increase the voltage slowly until vibration can just be felt. Average three measurements.

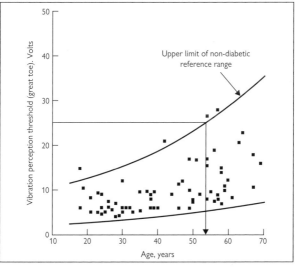

Figure 5.4 Vibration perception thresholds in non-diabetic subjects using the neurothesiometer at the great toe pulp (Levy 1992, unpublished data). Using a non-age-related threshold to predict high risk of progression to ulceration (e.g. 25 V as shown) will result in under-diagnosis of significant neuropathy in patients under ~55 years

Table 5.2 Autonomic function tests—reference ranges			
	Normal	Borderline	Abnormal
Heart rate variation to deep breathing (beats/min)	≥15	11–14	≤10
Systolic BP fall 2 min after standing (mmHg)	≤10	11–29	≥30

For routine clinical examination of the foot, a 2008 ADA/AACE report suggests the use of one, preferably two, of the following five tests to identify the high-risk foot: 10 g monofilament, 128 Hz tuning fork, pinprick sensation, ankle reflexes, and vibration perception threshold (Boulton et al. 2008).

5.5.4 Common syndromes of somatic neuropathy

5.5.4.1 Foot ulceration

Foot ulceration always involves advanced sensory neuropathy (often asymptomatic autonomic neuropathy as well), local tissue ischaemia caused by abnormal focal plantar pressures, and infection. In Type 1 diabetes, neuropathy is overwhelmingly more important than PVD in causing foot ulceration, unless there is advanced renal impairment, where PVD is common. Always request a plain radiograph of the foot to help diagnose osteomyelitis and Charcot neuroarthropathy (Box 5.7). Early radiological changes are uncommon, but pathology can become obvious within a short time, especially in a Charcot foot. Although a population study in Sweden found a reassuring fall in the number of non-traumatic lower limb amputations in Type 1 diabetes over the past decade, and they almost never occurred under 30 yrs of age, there is still an 80-fold increased risk compared with the non-diabetic population, and by age 65, men have a cumulative risk of about 20%, women 11% (Jonasson et al. 2008).

5.5.4.2 Charcot neuroarthropathy

A rapidly destructive arthropathy characteristic of Type 1 diabetes often associated with other advanced tissue complications. The cause is not known, and the neurophysiological findings in Charcot patients and those with recurrent foot ulceration are similar. Trauma and painless stress-type fractures (metatarsal shafts and bases) are frequent precipitants. Osteoclastic activity is markedly increased. Midfoot bones are usually involved, but metatarsophalangeal joints and rarely more proximal joints can be affected. It usually presents as a 'hot' foot in a patient without ulceration—though secondary ulceration caused by the mechanical disorganization of the foot is common. Always consider the diagnosis—early immobilization with total contact casting to stabilize the foot is important to slow progression.

> **Box 5.7 Key points in the management of neuropathic foot ulceration**
>
> - *Multidisciplinary team* is critical, especially podiatry, clinical microbiology, surgeon, and orthotist; low threshold for hospital admission, as symptoms are a poor indication of severity of infection.
> - *Exclude significant peripheral disease*: ankle-brachial pressure index – if reduced (<0.6–0.7), MRA with a view to revascularization
> - *Plain radiography*: osteomyelitis, early Charcot neuroarthropathy, asymptomatic fractures
> - *Relieve pressure*: bedrest, total contact casting/Aircast
> - *Debridement*: specialist podiatry, surgical (for abscesses and widespread necrosis), medical (larval)
> - *Antibiotics*: guided, where possible, by culture of deep specimens. Cover methicillin-resistant *Staphylococcus aureus* (MRSA) in patients with recurrent foot ulceration or frequent hospitalization. Always cover staphyloccoci and streptococci. Distal osteomyelitis of a digit often resolves with prolonged course of bone-penetrating antibiotics

Distinction from osteomyelitis is difficult (rarely they may co-exist) but a normal CRP or absence of current ulceration would be useful indicators of a Charcot process. MRI may show bone oedema, occult fractures, and joint effusions before changes are seen on plain radiographs. Bisphosphonates (pamidronate 90 mg as a single infusion) improves laboratory and clinical markers over 12 months, but the long-term outcomes are not known (Jude et al. 2001). Once the acute episode settles, assess for specialized footwear, and surgical stabilization may be considered.

5.4.3 *Peripheral mononeuropathies*

Carpal tunnel syndrome (CTS) is extremely common in Type 1 diabetes, affecting 85% of patients after 50 yrs or longer duration. Although independent of other microvascular complications, it is especially common in dialysis patients. The overall prevalence is ~20% (Singh et al. 2005). Consider the diagnosis whenever patients present with pain or ache in the hand or forearm, especially at night. Check thyroid function, remembering the association between Type 1 diabetes, hypothyroidism, and CTS. Request median nerve conduction study and refer for surgical assessment. Surgical outcome is variably reported as good as, or poorer than, non-diabetic subjects. The clinical impression is of a less satisfactory outcome in patients who may well have other hand abnormalities (see below). Proximal motor neuropathy (diabetic amyotrophy) and truncal neuropathies occasionally seen in Type 2 diabetes are very uncommon in Type 1 diabetes.

5.5.4.4 *Cranial mononeuropathies*

Painless, usually pupil-sparing third cranial nerve palsies, and sixth nerve palsies are not uncommon in long-standing Type 1 diabetes, with or without evidence of other microvascular complications. Lesions are thought to be focal microvascular thrombosis in capillaries supplying the peripheral course of the nerve, though midbrain MRI lesions have been found in some patients with third nerve lesions. They usually resolve spontaneously over several months, but require urgent ophthalmological and orthoptic input for correction of the severe diplopia. Patients over 50 should have a brain MRI scan.

5.5.4.5 *Cheiroarthropathy and the diabetic hand*

Although not purely neuropathic, it is worthwhile considering this common problem here. The disabled and stiff, but not usually painful, hand can occur in up to 35% of Type 1 patients, especially those with co-existing microvascular complications. The cheiroarthropathy itself is caused by thickening of the flexor tendon sheaths and subcutaneous tissues, giving the characteristic 'prayer sign'—a gap between the opposed raised hands. It frequently occurs together with:

- CTS
- Peripheral neuropathy
- Flexor tenosynovitis (trigger finger), often multiple
- Dupuytren's contracture (usually mild and non-progressive, involving the middle and ring fingers; Chammas *et al.* 1995).

Each component requires detailed assessment and individualized treatment. There may be an inflammatory element; there is a report of it rapidly resolving after pancreas transplantation with corticosteroid immunosuppression.

5.5.5 **Common syndromes of autonomic neuropathy**

5.5.5.1 *Gastroparesis and large bowel involvement*

Gastroparesis occurs most commonly in young people, especially women, with longstanding poorly controlled diabetes, and therefore may be associated with eating disorders (see Chapters 7 and 8). Other neuropathic complications, but interestingly not foot ulceration, are common. Consider it in the following situations:

- Abrupt worsening of glycaemic control, especially unexpected hypoglycaemia—mismatch between insulin injection and the delay of gastric contents moving into the small intestine
- Recurrent episodes of vomiting
- Recurrent diabetic ketoacidosis.

Symptoms are very variable, and may only be slight fullness during meals, early satiety, or postprandial hypoglycaemia. Later, episodic nausea, vomiting, weight loss, and malnutrition can occur. Upper gastrointestinal symptoms, though related to neuropathy, are poorly correlated with impaired gastric emptying. A formal gastric emptying study (half-time to empty isotope-labelled fluid and solid) should be performed, and frequently demonstrates delays of several hours; upper gastrointestinal endoscopy is usually done, and may demonstrate retained gastric contents, and co-existent gastroduodenal and oesophageal pathology. Autonomic function tests are useful, and near-absent heart-rate variation to deep breathing (vagal abnormality), even in these young patients, would be expected.

Medical treatment is unsatisfactory. Use fast-acting analogues and advise postprandial injection. Metoclopramide 5 to 10 mg tds (not in the under 20s), domperidone 10 to 20 mg tds before meals, and low-dose erythromycin suspension 125 mg tds should be tried. However, many of these patients require enteral feeding in the medium term to reduce recurrent hospital admissions, while considering:

- Gastric drainage procedure, for example gastroenterostomy with Roux loop
- Implantable gastric pacemaker
- Pancreatic or islet cell transplantation.

Constipation (large bowel atony) is common, and may alternate with diarrhoea, which is characteristically episodic, lasting a few days, then remitting, and nocturnal, sometimes associated with faecal incontinence. Consider other causes, for example malabsorption, coeliac disease, thyrotoxicosis; malignancy would be very rare in these mostly young patients. Symptomatic treatment is variably effective (codeine phosphate 30 mg or loperamide 2 mg tds-qds). For episodic diarrhoea, a 7- to 10-day course of oxytetracycline or erythromycin, 250 mg qds is sometimes successful, at least initially. Refractory diarrhoea may respond to subcutaneous octreotide or long-acting somatostatin analogues (Corbould and Campbell 2009).

5.5.5.2 Perioperative risks (see Section 3.5.2)
Established cardiovascular autonomic neuropathy is associated with a two- to threefold increased risk of intraoperative morbidity and mortality, possible contributions being haemodynamic instability and hypothermia. Alert anaesthetists to this risk in these apparently well younger people; aspiration of retained gastric contents during intubation as a result of severe but asymptomatic gastroparesis has been reported.

5.5.5.3 Symptomatic postural hypotension
Symptoms, frequently disabling, correlate poorly with postural BP changes. Because sympathetic autonomic neuropathy is late, these patients are often older than those with gastrointestinal symptoms, and frequently have other advanced microvascular complications, the treatment of which may make postural symptoms worse. Daytime

hypotension with recumbent hypertension (document with ABPM) can occur and is difficult to manage. Elastic stockings and raising the head of the bed 10 cm may help. Try to avoid all drugs that might worsen symptoms. The following drugs have been tried; there is trial data for fludrocortisone and midodrine:

- *Fludrocortisone*, starting at a low dose, for example 50 µg daily, with careful monitoring of electrolytes and BP for development or exacerbation of hypertension
- *DDAVP (desmopressin)* for example 0.1 mL nasal solution, or one dose of nasal spray (10 µg each). Monitor electrolytes frequently—there is a risk of hyponatraemia
- *Erythropoietin*, in close association with the nephrology team; the effect on BP may not simply be through increasing red cell mass (autonomic neuropathy may be associated with anaemia in the presence of normal renal function). Thrombotic and other risks preclude its use when haemoglobin >11 g/dL
- *Midodrine*, an α-agonist, is specifically indicated for neurogenic postural hypotension, but is not licensed in the UK.

5.5.5.4 *Erectile dysfunction (ED)*

ED is possibly even more common in Type 1 than Type 2 diabetes, with age-specific incidence increasing from 10% in the 21 to 29 yrs age group to nearly 50% in the over 40s, and from 16% in those with duration 11 to 14 yrs to 38% after more than 25 yrs (Klein *et al.* 2005). Endothelial dysfunction probably underlies ED in Type 1 diabetes as it does in Type 2, but the spectrum of vascular risk factors contributing to endothelial dysfunction may be different (dyslipidaemia and hypertension, for example, are likely to be less important). The introduction of three phosphodiesterase type 5 inhibitor drugs, prototype sildenafil, has revolutionized ED management. Type 1 patients benefited from sildenafil (the 100 mg dose was required in 70%), compared with placebo, independent of smoking status and glycaemic control, but patients with severe ED derived less benefit (Stuckey *et al.* 2003). Tadalafil and vardenafil are effective within about 30 min, sildenafil in about 1 h. The long-acting tadalafil, given daily in low dose (2.5 or 5 mg, compared with the standard single dose of 10 or 20 mg), is an effective alternative to on-demand dosing (Hatzichristou *et al.* 2008).

5.5.6 **Medical treatment of diabetic polyneuropathy**

Despite more than 20 yrs of intensive clinical investigation, no specific adjuvant drug treatment other than good glycaemic control has been shown to benefit diabetic polyneuropathy. The aldose reductase inhibitor epalrestat is available in some parts of the world, but clinical trial results of this class have been disappointing, either through lack of efficacy or adverse effects. The antioxidant α-lipoic acid may have some beneficial effects, but again is not licensed in the UK. The protein kinase C β-inhibitor ruboxistaurin, whose primary value is in retinopathy, has shown minor and generally disappointing results in neuropathy, and the seemingly logical nerve growth factor is ineffective. Nerve conduction measurements improved slightly after co-administration of C-peptide together with usual insulin, indicating that C-peptide is not a redundant molecule but may be bioactive.

5.6 Microvascular complications in very longstanding Type 1 diabetes (>50 yrs)

Two large populations of people surviving more than 50 yrs of Type 1 diabetes have been reported, one in the UK and the other in the USA. Their clinical characteristics (Table 5.3) are startlingly similar. In particular they are phenotypically insulin-sensitive, requiring low insulin doses, with a low body mass index (BMI), extremely high high-density lipoprotein (HDL) cholesterol levels, and low triglycerides (HDL and triglycerides—but not total or LDL cholesterol, or, surprisingly, A1C—were nearly uniformly statistically significantly different between those with and without any microvascular complications). In addition, in the USA cohort, current exercise was strongly protective against complications, and in the UK cohort, moderate alcohol consumption—both characteristics whose effects may be mediated via HDL cholesterol. The near-50% male: female split and the longevity of the subjects' parents are striking, and hint strongly at protective genetic or familial factors, despite over 60% of the UK group being current or ex-smokers. Only about 50% of the USA patients reported retinopathy, contrasting with the widespread view that nearly all patients will have retinopathy after 20 to 30 yrs duration, and this proportion continued to fall with increasing duration beyond 50 yrs. Both populations had low prevalences of diabetic nephropathy, though 36% of the UK group had micro- or macroalbuminuria. While these are not longitudinal studies, it seems unlikely that any of the factors identified at 50+ yrs will have been significantly different in the remote past—especially, of course, HDL cholesterol levels, which are effectively unmodifiable. The mechanisms by which very high HDL cholesterol protect against microvascular complications are not known, though it is tempting to believe it is due to powerful non-lipid characteristics of HDL cholesterol, for example its intriguing anti-inflammatory actions. High HDL cholesterol may be a reliable indicator of a good prognosis even shortly after diagnosis.

CHAPTER 5 Microvascular complications

Table 5.3 Characteristics of long survivors (>50 yrs) of Type 1 diabetes on both sides of the Atlantic (Bain et al. 2003; Keenan et al. 2007)

	UK Golden Years Cohort (2003)	USA 50-yr Medalist Study (2007)
Age, yrs	69	70
Age at onset, yrs	13.7 Mean duration 56 yrs	12.6
Number studied, % male	400, 54%	326, 45%
BMI	25.0	24.5
A1C at examination (%)	7.6%	7.0%
Insulin dose (U/kg/day)	0.52	0.5
HDL cholesterol, mmol/L	1.84	1.85 (no microvascular complications) 1.67 (microvascular complications)
Triglycerides, mmol/L	1.5 (non-fasting)	0.8 (no microvascular complications) 1.0 (microvascular complications)
Family history: mean age of parents' death, yrs	72 (fathers and mothers)	74 (fathers) 78 (mothers)—compare mean life expectancy for this birth cohort (~1900)—48 yrs

References

94

ACE Inhibitors in Diabetic Nephropathy Trialist Group (2001). Should all patients with type 1 diabetes mellitus and microalbuminuria receive angiotensin-converting enzyme inhibitors? *Ann Intern Med*, **134**: 370–9. [PMID: 11242497]

Amin R, Widmer B, Prevost AT et al. (2008). Risk of microalbuminuria and progression to macroalbuminuria in a cohort with childhood onset type 1 diabetes: prospective observational study. *BMJ*, **336**: 697–701. [PMID: 18349042]

Bain SC, Gill GV, Dyer PH et al. (2003). Characteristics of Type 1 diabetes of over 50 years duration (the Golden Years Cohort). *Diabet Med*, **20**: 808–11. [PMID: 14510860]

Bloom S, Till, S, Sonksen P, Smith S (1984). Use of a biothesiometer to measure individual vibration thresholds and their variation in 519 non-diabetic subjects. *BMJ*, **288**: 1793–5. [PMID: 6428547]

Boulton AJ, Vinik AI, Arezzo JC et al.; American Diabetes Association (2008). Diabetic neuropathies. *Diabetes Care*, **28**: 956–62. [PMID: 15793206]

Brownlee M (2005). The pathobiology of diabetic complications: a unifying mechanism. *Diabetes*, **54**: 1615–25. [PMID: 15919781]

Chammas M, Bousquet P, Renard EM, Poirier JL, Jaffiol C, Allieu Y (1995). Dupuytren's disease, carpal tunnel syndrome, trigger finger, and diabetes mellitus. *J Hand Surg [Am]*, **20**: 109–14. [PMID: 7722249]

Chaturvedi N, Sjoelie AK, Porta M *et al.* (2001). Markers of insulin resistance are strong risk factors for retinopathy incidence in type 1 diabetes. *Diabetes Care*, **24**: 284–9. [PMID: 11213880]

Chaturvedi N, Porta M, Klein R *et al.*; for the DIRECT Programme Study Group (2008). Effect of candesartan on prevention (DIRECT-Prevent 1) and progression (DIRECT-Protect 1) of retinopathy in type 1 diabetes: randomised, placebo-controlled trials. *Lancet*, **372**: 1394–402. [PMID: 18823656]

Corbould A, Campbell J (2009). Efficacy of octreotide but not long-acting somatostatin analogue for severe refractory diabetic diarrhoea. *Diabet Med*, **26**: 828–9. [PMID: 19701956]

Costacou T, Ellis D, Fried L, Orchard TJ (2007). Sequence of progression of albuminuria and decreased GFR in persons with type 1 diabetes: a cohort study. *Am J Kidney Dis*, **50**: 721–32. [PMID: 17954285]

Diabetes Control and Complications Trial Research Group (1993). The effect of intensive treatment of diabetes on the development and progression of long-term complications in insulin-dependent diabetes mellitus. *N Engl J Med*, **329**: 977–86. [PMID: 8366922]

Diabetes Control and Complications Trial Research Group (1995a). Implementation of treatment protocols in the Diabetes Control and Complications Trial. *Diabetes Care*, **18**: 361–76. [PMID: 7555480]

Diabetes Control and Complications Trial Research Group (1995b). The effect of intensive diabetes therapy on the development and progression of neuropathy. *Ann Intern Med*, **122**: 561–8. [PMID: 7887548]

Diabetes Control and Complications Trial Research Group (1996). The absence of a glycemic threshold for the development of long-term complications: the perspective of the Diabetes Control and Complications Trial. *Diabetes*, **45**: 1289–98. [PMID: 8826962]

Diabetes Control and Complications Trial Research Group (1998). Effect of intensive therapy on residual β-cell function in patients with type 1 diabetes in the Diabetes Control and Complications Trial. *Ann Intern Med*, **128**: 517–23. [PMID: 9518395]

Diabetes Control and Complications Trial Research Group/Epidemiology of Diabetes Interventions and Complications Research Group. (2000). Retinopathy and nephropathy in patients with Type 1 diabetes four years after a trial of intensive therapy. *N Engl J Med*, **342**: 381–9. [PMID: 1066428]

Feldman EL, Stevens MJ, Thomas PK, Brown MB, Canal N, Greene DA (1994). A practical two-step quantitative clinical and electrophysiological assessment for the diagnosis and staging of diabetic neuropathy. *Diabetes Care*, **17**: 1281–9. [PMID: 7821168]

Hatzichristou D, Gambla M, Rubio-Aurioles E *et al.* (2008). Efficacy of tadalafil once daily in men with diabetes mellitus and erectile dysfunction. *Diabet Med*, **25**: 138–46. [PMID: 18290855]

Jonasson JM, Ye W, Sparén P, Apelqvist J, Nyrén O, Brismar K (2008). Risks of nontraumatic lower-extremity amputations in patients with type 1 diabetes: a population-based cohort study in Sweden. *Diabetes Care*, **31**: 1536–40. [PMID: 18443192]

Jude EB, Selby PL, Burgess J *et al.* (2001). Bisphosphonates in the treatment of Charcot neuroarthopathy: a double-blind randomised controlled trial. *Diabetologia*, **44**: 2032–7. [PMID: 11719835]

Keenan HA, Costacou T, Sun HK *et al.* (2007). Clinical factors associated with resistance to microvascular complications in diabetic patients of extreme disease duration: the 50-year medalist study. *Diabetes Care*, **30**: 1995–7. [PMID: 17507696]

Klein R, Klein BE, Moss SE *et al.* (1984). The Wisconsin epidemiologic study of diabetic retinopathy. II. Prevalence and risk of diabetic retinopathy when age at diagnosis is less than 30 years. *Arch Ophthalmol*, **102**: 520–6. [PMID: 6367724]

Klein R, Klein BE, Moss SE (2005). Ten-year incidence of self-reported erectile dysfunction in people with long-term type 1 diabetes. *J Diabetes Complications*, **19**: 35–41. [PMID: 15642488]

Lewis EJ, Hunsucker LG, Bain RP, Rohde RD (1993). The effect of angiotensin-converting enzyme inhibition on diabetic nephropathy. *N Engl J Med*, **329**: 1456–62. [PMID: 8413456]

Malone JI, Morrison AD, Pavan PR, Cuthbertson DD (2001). Prevalence and significance of retinopathy in subjects with type 1 diabetes of less than 5 years' duration screened for the diabetes control and complications trial. *Diabetes Care*, **24**: 522–6. [PMID: 11289479]

Mann JF, Schmeider RE, McQueen M *et al.* (2008). Renal outcomes with telmisartan, ramipril, or both, in people at high vascular risk (the ONTARGET study): a multicentre, randomised, double-blind, controlled trial. *Lancet*, **372**: 547–53. [PMID: 18707986]

Martin CL, Albers J, Herman WH *et al.* (2006). Neuropathy among the Diabetes Control and Complications Trial cohort 8 years after trial completion. *Diabetes Care*, **29**: 340–4. [PMID: 16443884]

Mauer M, Zinman B, Gardiner R *et al.* (2009). Renal and retinal effects of enalapril and losartan in type 1 diabetes. *N Engl J Med*, **361**: 40–51. [PMID: 19571282]

Mohsin F, Craig ME, Cusumano J *et al.* (2005). Discordant trends in microvascular complications in adolescents with type 1 diabetes from 1990 to 2002. *Diabetes Care*, **28**: 1974–80. [PMID: 16043741]

Nordwall M, Bojestig M, Arnqvist JH, Ludvigsson J; Linköping Diabetes Complications Study (2004). Declining incidence of severe retinopathy and persisting decrease of nephropathy in an unselected population of Type 1 diabetes—the Linköping Diabetes Complications Study. *Diabetologia*, **47**: 1266–72. [PMID: 15235723]

Perkins BA, Ficociello LH, Silva KH, Finkelstein DM, Warram JH, Kro-lewski AS (2003). Regression of microalbuminuria in type 1 diabetes. *N Engl J Med*, **348**: 2285–93. [PMID: 12788992]

Rossing P (2005). The changing epidemiology of diabetic microangiopathy in type 1 diabetes. *Diabetologia*, **48**: 1439–44. [PMID: 15986235]

Schjoedt KJ, Hansen HP, Tarnow L, Rossing P, Parving HH (2008). Long-term prevention of diabetic nephropathy: an audit. *Diabetologia*, **51**: 956–61. [PMID: 18385971]

Singh R, Gamble G, Cundy T (2005). Lifetime risk of symptomatic carpal tunnel syndrome in type 1 diabetes. *Diabet Med*, **22**: 625–30. [PMID: 15842519]

Skrivarhaug T, Fosmark DS, Stene LC et al. (2006). Low cumulative inci-dence of proliferative retinopathy in childhood-onset type 1 diabetes: a 24-year follow-up study. *Diabetologia*, **49**: 2281–90. [PMID: 16955208]

Stuckey BG, Jadzinsky MN, Murphy LJ et al. (2003). Sildenafil citrate for treatment of erectile dysfunction in men with type 1 diabetes: results of a randomized controlled trial. *Diabetes Care*, **26**: 279–84. [PMID: 12547849]

Wright AD, Dodson PM (2010). Diabetic retinopathy and blockade of the renin-angiotensin: new data from the DIRECT study programme. *Eye (Lond)*, **24**: 1–6. [PMID: 19648902]

Zerbini G, Bonfati R, Meschi F et al. (2006). Persistent renal hypertrophy and faster decline of glomerular filtration rate precede the develop-ment of microalbuminuria in type 1 diabetes. *Diabetes*, **55**: 2620–5. [PMID: 16936212]

Further reading

Bennett MI (ed) (2006). *Neuropathic Pain (Oxford Pain Management Library)*. Oxford University Press, ISBN: 978-0-19-921569-0

Dodson PM (ed) (2008). *Diabetic retinopathy: screening to treatment (Oxford Diabetes Library)*. Oxford University Press, ISBN: 978-0-19-954496-7.

Donaghue KC, Chiarelli F, Trotta D, Allgrove J, Dahl-Jorgensen K (2007). ISPAD clinical practice consensus guidelines 2006–2007. Microvascular and macrovascular complications. *Pediatr Diabetes*, **8**: 163–70. [PMID: 17550427]

Fong DS, Aiello L, Gardner TW et al.; American Diabetes Association (2003). Diabetic retinopathy. *Diabetes Care*, **26** (Suppl 1): S99–102. [PMID: 12502630]

Tesfaye S, Boulton A (eds) (2009). *Diabetic neuropathy (Oxford Diabetes Library)*. Oxford University Press, ISBN: 978-0-19-955106-4.

Chapter 6

Macrovascular complications and lipids

Key points

- Premature macrovascular disease, especially coronary artery disease, is common in Type 1 diabetes, even in the absence of albuminuria.
- Stroke and peripheral vascular disease are also significantly more common.
- Hyperglycaemia is the most important risk factor, and clinical macrovascular events and surrogates (coronary calcification and carotid intima–media thickness) were less severe in the previous intensively treated Diabetes Control and Complications Trial (DCCT) cohort studied in Epidemiology of Diabetes Interventions and Complications (EDIC).
- In the absence of nephropathy, conventional lipid profiles in Type 1 patients are no different from those of non-diabetic individuals.
- There is no convincing evidence base for the routine use of statin treatment or low-dose aspirin in younger patients without complications.
- Insulin resistance, acquired through intensive insulin treatment and its associated weight gain, may contribute to macrovascular endpoints.

6.1 Introduction

Macrovascular disease—coronary artery disease (CAD), cerebro-vascular disease, and peripheral vascular disease (PVD)—is common and severe in Type 1 diabetes, but can be difficult to diagnose, and has been relatively ignored compared with the microvascular complications. This is strange, because first, cardiovascular (CV) mortality accounts for the majority of deaths in middle-aged Type 1 patients; second, atherosclerosis is undoubtedly accelerated (by at least 10 to 15 yrs in men, even more in women—the median age at first CV event in the Pittsburgh epidemiological study was just under 40 yrs); and third, the evidence for glycaemic control from the Diabetes Control and Complications Trial (DCCT) and Epidemiology of Diabetes

Interventions and Complications (EDIC) is at least as striking for macrovascular as for microvascular complications. Even old studies indicated that CAD was more frequent in Type 1 than Type 2 diabetes, and more recent studies confirm that the risk is at least similar for a given duration of follow-up, as well as indicating a stronger link between A1C and coronary risk (Juutilainen et al. 2008).

Because of the very strong link between diabetic nephropathy and CAD, and because nephropathy previously frequently occurred at an early age, this was thought to be the main causative link. However, nephropathy rates in Type 1 diabetes have fallen substantially over the past few decades, while CAD has not. Inflammatory factors (e.g. C-reactive protein (CRP), interleukin-6, PAI-1) may explain some of the excess CV risk. Females have an increased mortality. In the Diabetes UK cohort of patients diagnosed under 30 yrs of age, standardized mortality rate for CV mortality was 4.0 in women and 2.7 in men, but for ischaemic heart disease the ratios were even higher, and more disparate—8.8 in women, 4.5 in men (Laing et al. 1999). Most studies confirm the loss of premenopausal protection against CAD in women with Type 1, as in Type 2, diabetes (Box 6.1).

Box 6.1 Case history—extensive macrovascular disease in longstanding Type 1 diabetes

A Caucasian female was diagnosed in 1963 aged 28. A1C levels were usually between 8% and 9%, total cholesterol 5.7 to 6.3 mmol/L, HDL cholesterol 2.8 (side effects with statins), normal renal function, low-grade microalbuminuria (~60 mg/24 h), laser-treated proliferative retinopathy 1999. Persistently normotensive (<140/70). A pacemaker was inserted in 2004, at age 70, for slow atrial fibrillation; electrocardiogram (ECG) showed an old (silent) anteroseptal myocardial infarction. She had continuing shortness of breath, but no angina. Coronary angiography in 2006 showed diffuse atheroma and poor left ventricular function. At coronary bypass surgery in 2006, there was widespread palpable calcific arterial disease. Triple vessel bypass was performed, including internal mammary artery bypass to the only soft (mid) portion of the left anterior descending artery. She needed perioperative inotropic support, and had a postoperative ventricular fibrillation arrest. Hospital stay was 3 weeks. She died suddenly, 2 days after an uncomplicated routine incisional hernia repair 17 months later. At autopsy there were lacunar basal ganglia infarcts, a congested and fibrotic liver, and an old renal infarct. The aorta and carotid arteries were sclerotic with ulcerated calcific plaques; the right external iliac was obstructed by fibrocalcific plaques. The coronary grafts were patent, but the obtuse marginal branch was nearly obstructed after the bypass insertion point.

6.2 **Arterial changes**

6.2.1 **Early changes**

Arterial disease starts early in the course of Type 1 diabetes. Hyperglycaemia must be the major driving force at this stage, and the mechanisms postulated for glucose-mediated microvascular damage are presumed to be largely the same for large-vessel disease. Surrogate markers of arterial disease become abnormal early on:

* *Increased carotid intima–media thickness (CIMT)*, a reliable indicator of long-term coronary risk, has been found in children, adolescents, and young people with relatively short diabetes duration (Rabago Rodriguez *et al.* 2007).
* *Increased arterial stiffness* in peripheral (brachial, femoral, and carotid) and central vessels (aorta). Various non-invasive measures, including arterial elasticity and compliance, increased pulse wave velocity, reflecting arterial stiffness, and augmentation index, are abnormal in Type 1 diabetes, but the simplest measurement, increased systolic blood pressure, can be detected in patients in their 20s and 30s (Section 7.5.1) (Stehouwer *et al.* 2008).
* *Endothelial function* is also abnormal in early Type 1 diabetes even when CIMT is normal (Hurks *et al.* 2009). Various mechanisms are responsible, including, among others, decreased nitric oxide-induced vasodilatation, and increased vasoconstriction through endothelin-1 and angiotensin II, probably enhanced by glucose-activated inflammatory gene and NF-κB expression. Poor vitamin C status may also contribute.
* *Conventional arterial risk factors*: smoking, hypertension, and lipids.

6.2.2 **Later changes**

Hyperglycaemia is an ever-present factor behind atherosclerotic changes, but other pathogenic factors are likely to be involved. These include:

* *Cardiac autonomic neuropathy*. Abnormal heart rate variation and BP responses (see Chapter 5), and impaired perception of ischaemic cardiac pain, possibly contributing to silent coronary ischaemia
* *Microalbuminuria and proteinuria*. The Steno hypothesis proposes that microalbuminuria is a reliable indicator of the presence of widespread endothelial dysfunction. Microalbuminuria is associated with approximately one- to twofold increased risk of CV death, increasing to approximately tenfold (up to 40-fold in certain studies) in Type 1 patients with proteinuria. However, epidemiological and interventional studies (DCCT/EDIC) have described a persistent impact of hyperglycaemia even after controlling for proteinuric status.

6.3 **The scale of the problem—clinical studies**

6.3.1 **Coronary artery disease**

A few studies using methods to quantify CAD are now available. For example, the Oslo study investigated asymptomatic Type 1 patients, mean age 43 yrs, with a mean duration of 30 yrs (Larsen et al. 2002); the results fit with the Pittsburgh epidemiological data:

- 15% had abnormal exercise tolerance tests
- 34% had >50% stenosis in one or more main coronary arteries
- 10% (3 of 29) had triple vessel disease.

In a slightly different group, also without symptoms (mean age 52 yrs, duration 25 yrs) 22% had positive investigations, but only one patient had a positive exercise test; the remainder had a positive myocardial perfusion scan. A negative exercise test is therefore little reassurance of the absence of significant CAD, in these patients with diffuse, asymptomatic, but often extensive arterial disease (see Box 6.1).

Coronary calcification, detected by electron beam computed tomography (CT) scanning, can be performed in much larger groups of patients, and is a strong correlate of clinical CAD in Type 1 diabetes, especially in men. In DCCT/EDIC, men had consistently higher rates of any (>0) and significant (>200) coronary calcification Agatston scores than women, in both the intensive and conventional groups (Cleary et al. 2006).

6.3.2 **Cerebrovascular disease**

Again, a rather neglected area. In a large UK study (Laing et al. 2003) cerebrovascular disease accounted for 6% of all deaths, and 8% of deaths over the age of 40. Mortality was particularly high in women under 40. Most events were ischaemic, but there was a hint that haemorrhagic stroke was also increased. Strikingly, overall stroke mortality is similar to that in Type 2 diabetes. Not surprisingly, stroke risk increases tenfold in patients with nephropathy.

6.3.3 **Peripheral vascular disease**

Studies are hampered by poor definitions of PVD. There is a weak association between lower extremity calcification and coronary artery calcium scores. In addition to the CAD risk factors, autonomic neuropathy, consistently linked with vascular calcification, is an important factor (but note the Monckeberg's medial sclerosis characteristic of lower limb arterial calcification differs from the intimal calcification that develops in the coronaries).

6.4 **Identification of CAD in asymptomatic patients**

There is no agreed protocol for CAD screening in Type 2 patients, so it is not surprising that the problem in Type 1 patients has barely been addressed, despite the evidently high prevalence. Because of the very high rate of obstructive disease in patients with end-stage renal disease (ESRD), patients generally undergo coronary angiography before renal transplantation. In other groups, there is no consensus on the best screening tests, even those with high prior likelihood of CAD. High rates (>40%) of obstructive CAD were found on routine angiography in patients being considered for islet transplantation using the Edmonton protocol (these patients had very long duration, 27 to 35 yrs even at a relatively young age, 42 to 49 yrs), but standard exercise stress testing and myocardial perfusion imaging (MPI) had low sensitivity. However, in clinical practice, an initial combination of non-invasive tests, according to local availability, should be considered (exercise stress testing, myocardial perfusion scanning, stress echocardiography, CT for coronary calcification, cardiac MRI). Evidence-based clinical guidelines are urgently needed.

6.4.1 **Risk prediction**

Risk prediction models as validated and used in Type 2 diabetes, for example Framingham and UKPDS, are unlikely to be valid for Type 1 diabetes. Confounding factors include on the one hand the longer duration of glycaemic exposure, the lower age at which CHD events occur in Type 1 patients, the profound impact of nephropathy, and on the other hand the lower rates of hypertension and dyslipidaemia in the absence of nephropathy. The UKPDS risk engine markedly underestimated the risk of CHD events in the Pittsburgh cohort, and not surprisingly, since it contained very few people with diabetes, let alone Type 1 diabetes, the Framingham risk model exhibited 'lack of calibration' in males and females alike (Zgibor et al. 2006).

Until an appropriate risk equation is developed, therefore, a risk-factor approach suggests considering screening asymptomatic patients with poorly controlled long-standing Type 1 diabetes (e.g. 20 yrs or more adult duration), those with established microvascular complications, especially microalbuminuria, and those with multiple conventional risk factors (smoking, hypertension, hyperlipidaemia; Box 6.2).

6.5 **DCCT/EDIC—glycaemic control and CV disease**

During the 6.5 yrs DCCT follow-up intensive treatment was associated with non-significantly fewer CV events (23 vs 40), but by the end

103

Box 6.2 Factors associated with CAD and its progression in Type 1 diabetes

- *Associated factors*
  - Diabetes duration
  - Body mass index, waist–hip ratio
  - Albumin excretion rate
  - Glycaemic control
  - Smoking, hypertension, hypercholesterolaemia, non-high density LDL
  - Coronary calcification Agatston score (>100, >400)
- *Factors associated with progression*
  - Increase in BMI
  - ?Glycaemic control
  - ?High insulin dose and dose per body weight
  - BP
  - Serum triglycerides and cholesterol
  - ?Elevated white blood cell count

of the total 17 yrs total follow-up in EDIC, although the ratio of events was similar (46 vs 98; 57% risk reduction), the difference had become statistically highly significant, and remained so after correction for microalbuminuria and proteinuria. An A1C reduction of 10% was associated with 20% reduction in CV event rate. The proportions of both silent and symptomatic myocardial infarction, known to have similar prognostic significance, were broadly the same in the two treatment groups. There were no differences in medication between the two groups that could have affected the results (The DCCT/EDIC Study Group 2005). Because glycaemic control was similar in the two groups during 11 yrs of EDIC, it is clear that:

- Glycaemic control is the most important factor in determining macrovascular outcomes in Type 1 diabetes.
- As with microvascular complications, it is important to optimize glycaemic control as soon as possible after diagnosis.

6.5.1 Surrogate measures of cardiac risk

6.5.1.1 *Carotid intima–media thickness*

CIMT was no different from that of non-diabetic controls at the beginning of EDIC (contrasting with many studies, even some in children and adolescents; see Section 7.6). By year 6 of EDIC (13 yrs total follow-up, mean diabetes duration ~18 yrs, mean age late 30s) diabetic patients had developed increased CIMT, which increased more slowly in the intensive group. Nearly all the differences in CIMT were explained by the differences in A1C during DCCT, but follow-up was not long enough to determine whether this was associated with CV event reduction (Nathan et al. 2003).

6.5.1.2 Coronary calcification

Patients were scanned at EDIC years 7 to 9 (16 yrs total follow-up, mean duration ~21 yrs, mean age nearly 43 yrs, BMI 28). Clinically significant scores (>200 Agatston units) were less prevalent (7%) in the intensive group compared with the conventional group (10%), with glycaemia during the DCCT accounting for much of the difference (Cleary et al. 2006). As with CIMT, it was a cross-sectional study, so the relationship between progression of coronary calcification and events in the groups could not be analysed. CIMT and coronary artery calcification (CAC) score are both relatively simple and reproducible measurements, though CT scanning involves significant irradiation, but analysis of CAC scores is complicated by their highly skewed distribution (e.g. in the EDIC study up to 78% of the intensive group and 65% of the conventional group had zero calcification). In addition, there is lack of agreement for criterion CAC scores for significant obstructive disease (various studies use scores of 100, 200 (EDIC), or 400).

6.6 Lipids

6.6.1 Lipid profiles and glycaemic control

Very poor glycaemic control is often associated with elevated LDL and triglycerides and depressed HDL levels, probably due to impaired lipoprotein lipase activity. However, the conventional lipid profile of type 1 patients in stable control and without microvascular complications, especially microalbuminuria, is identical to that of non-diabetic people, so the contribution of lipids to their premature atheroma is not clear. Subtle alterations in lipoproteins have been described that may be of importance (see below).

The best data on stable lipid profiles comes from the DCCT/EDIC (Jenkins et al. 2003). Mean measurements in the DCCT baseline lipid profile were:

Total cholesterol	4.6 mmol/L
Triglycerides	0.9 mmol/L
HDL cholesterol	1.3 mmol/L
LDL cholesterol	2.8 mmol/L

with HDL, as expected, higher in women than men, and triglycerides slightly lower. Interestingly, at the end of DCCT these profiles had barely changed, and there were no clinically significant differences between the intensive and conventional groups (no patients were taking lipid-lowering treatment at the end of DCCT (1993)–4S, the first major lipid intervention study using a statin did not report until 1994). By year 11 of EDIC, triglycerides had slightly increased, as had

105

HDL cholesterol, but LDL was unchanged, despite around one-third of patients in both previous intensive and conventional groups taking statins by this time. Other studies in pump-treated patients have reported more obvious decrease in triglycerides, and in total and LDL cholesterol with A1C reductions from 9% to 7%—approximately the change in the intensive DCCT group. In the subgroup of intensively treated DCCT patients who did not gain weight, a factor driving lipid profiles towards a more insulin-resistant picture, small changes occurred in the expected direction (e.g. LDL decreased from 2.8 to 2.7 mmol/L, HDL increased from 1.26 to 1.40 mmol/L).

In the DCCT/EDIC, detailed lipid analyses, including nuclear magnetic resonance profiles, uncovered many slight adverse qualitative changes in men compared with women, for example higher LDL concentrations, lower levels of large (good) HDL, higher levels of small (bad) HDL, and overall smaller HDL particles, together with higher concentrations of total atherogenic particles (apoB) and triglycerides, and lower levels of protective apoA1-associated particles. These were weakly associated with glycaemic control, and some were cross sectionally associated with CIMT. However, importantly, these gender differences were not reflected in the CV endpoints—equal numbers of males and females had events, confirming again the obliteration of female premenopausal protection against CV events in diabetes. The abnormal HDL pattern was also found in the EURODIAB study, but there was no association with coronary calcification score. Other factors involved in lipid metabolism may be involved, for example cholesteryl ester transfer protein (CETP) lecithin cholesterol acyl transferase (LCAT), and paraoxonase—the last is associated with HDL particles, and can retard lipoprotein oxidation while metabolizing oxidized lipids (Levy and Galton 2005). It is difficult to determine what contribution these abnormalities make to the markedly increased atherogenesis seen in Type 1 diabetes (perhaps multiple minor abnormalities sustained over a long period have a significant cumulative effect), and whether early intervention will have a clinically important effect.

More important therapeutically, Type 1 patients tend to have increased cholesterol absorption and decreased synthesis compared with Type 2 patients, possibly because of ineffective insulin action leading to down-regulation of enterocyte cholesterol transport mechanisms. This may explain the relative effectiveness of the cholesterol absorption inhibitor ezetimibe.

6.6.2 **Lipids and diabetic nephropathy**

Lipid abnormalities increase with progressing proteinuria, and are especially marked in the nephrotic syndrome. These include:

Increased total and LDL cholesterol, due to decreased LDL catabolism. There is an inverse relationship between serum albumin and total and LDL cholesterol

Low or normal HDL levels

Elevated triglycerides.

The importance of albuminuria can be seen from the relatively normal lipid profiles of non-nephrotic patients with chronic kidney disease (CKD) stages 2 to 4, whether or not they have diabetes. However, LDL levels tend to be higher in haemo- and peritoneal dialysis patients, and after transplantation antirejection drugs can also be associated with elevated LDL (Molitch 2006). There is some evidence that dyslipidaemia, especially low HDL, is a risk factor for decreased renal function after correction for other known risk factors, and LDL, oxidized in mesangial cells, can lead to cell injury and vasoconstriction. Though separate data were not presented for Type 1 patients in the Heart Protection Study (2003), simvastatin 40 mg daily for 5 yrs reduced the rate of decline of eGFR in the whole diabetes cohort.

6.7 Lipid management and aspirin therapy

7.1 Lipids

While there is no evidence for the benefit of routine lipid-lowering treatment in Type 1 patients under 40 who have no evidence of microvascular complications and no other macrovascular risk factors, guidelines, while acknowledging the lack of evidence, nevertheless propose it. The Heart Protection Study reports tantalizingly little detail about the small cohort (615, 10%) of Type 1 patients, but it appears to offer little evidence for treatment of this group. They had a very long duration of diabetes (mean 29 yrs), and their mean age was presumably similar to that of the Type 2 cohort (62 yrs), with a high proportion of vascular complications. Overall macrovascular events were 7% to 8% less frequent than in the Type 2 group but absolute and relative risk reductions with simvastatin treatment (~4%, 22%, respectively) were similar. Similar limited conclusions can be reached from a meta-analysis of nearly 1500 Type 1 patients in 14 RCTs, from 4S (1994) to CARDS (2004), though most of the trials contained trivial numbers of Type 1, compared with Type 2, patients (Cholesterol Treatment Trialists' Collaborators 2008). Nearly 50% of the Type 1 patients had previous vascular events and hypertension; their lipid profile was similar to that of the Type 2 patients in the same study total cholesterol 5.7, LDL 3.4, HDL 1.3, triglycerides slightly lower than the Type 2 patients—1.6 vs 2.1 mmol/L). Their similarity to the

Type 2 patients would certainly warrant statin treatment; they clearly differ from the DCCT/EDIC patients (Section 6.6.1).

Patients with any risk factors that would warrant treatment Type 2 diabetes should have statin treatment. These include:

- Hypertension, for example >140/80 (or treated hypertension), with or without microalbuminuria
- Multiple manifestations of the metabolic syndrome (see below)
- Any microvascular complications (including neuropathy)
- Smoking.

Before considering pharmacological treatment, dietary management should be reinforced, and non-pharmacological agents considered. Plant stanols at the recommended dose of 2 g/day may reduce LDL cholesterol by up to 16% in Type 1 patients, and fish oils may have particular benefits in reducing atherogenic apoB-containing particles. Thereafter, the decision to start statin treatment in patients without more clear-cut indications must be individualized, especially younger uncomplicated patients with short diabetes duration and those with LDL levels <3 mmol/L; where available, CIMT and coronary calcification scores could usefully be included in the clinical decision-making process. Again, RCT evidence is urgently needed.

Once the decision to start treatment has been made, LDL targets should be the same as those in Type 2 patients, that is <2 mmol/L patients without evidence of vascular disease, and considerably lower, <1.7 to 1.8 mmol/L where there is. Simvastatin titrated up to 4 mg nocte, followed by either a more potent statin or addition of ezetimibe 10 mg daily, as in Type 2 patients, would be appropriate. While ezetimibe may be very effective in LDL lowering in Type 1 patients, there is no evidence for a beneficial effect on CV event reduction, and there is concern about efficacy.

6.7.2 Aspirin

There are similar controversies and uncertainties over low-dose aspirin treatment in primary prevention. The American Diabetes Association recommendation is identical for both Type 1 and Type 2 diabetes: consider low-dose aspirin (75 to 162 mg daily) in patients over the age of 40, or those with an additional CV risk factor (family history of CVD, hypertension, smoking, dyslipidaemia, and albuminuria). However, the level of evidence is much lower in Type 1 diabetes and there is currently no evidence for its use in patients with no additional risk factors, even in those with long duration diabetes. Patients with retinopathy, micro- or macroalbuminuria should probably take aspirin because of the significantly increased CV risk associated with these complications.

6.8 **Metabolic syndrome and Type 1 diabetes**

About 15% of Type 1 patients can be formally classified as having the metabolic syndrome, increasing to about 30% in those with diabetes duration of 20 yrs or longer. Increased macrovascular events have been described in longitudinal studies, but the same caveats must be applied to Type 1 patients as all others with the metabolic syndrome: for example, in the Pittsburgh study the individual components of the metabolic syndrome (using any of the formal definitions) better predicted major diabetes outcomes than the full syndrome, but, perhaps not surprisingly, microalbuminuria was by far the most powerful predictor, conferring a hazard ratio of 9 for mortality and 6 for a combined measure of clinically important outcomes—CAD, renal failure, and diabetes-related death (Pambianco et al. 2007).

Type 1 patients with a family history of Type 2 diabetes have several insulin-resistant characteristics, but it is the modifiable causes of acquired insulin resistance that are of greater practical interest. The majority of patients in the DCCT gained weight throughout the trial, with the intensively treated group gaining the most. Overweight increased from 12% to 17% in the conventional treatment group, and from 19% to 34% in the intensive group (DCCT Research Group 1995). The intensive group with the highest quartile of weight gain was clinically obese, with a mean BMI of 31 kg/m^2. This was associated with a deteriorating lipid profile (increased total and LDL cholesterol, and apoB) and slightly increased systolic, but not diastolic blood pressure. Perhaps unexpectedly, there were no changes in triglycerides or HDL, despite increased intra-abdominal fat. In short, intensive treatment induces a mild insulin-resistant state. High-sensitivity CRP (hsCRP) was higher in the DCCT/EDIC prior intensive group than the conventional group, and related to features of the metabolic syndrome, especially BMI and waist–hip ratio, and also oral contraceptive use and female gender. However, there was no association between hsCRP and complications.

6.8.1 **Polycystic ovarian syndrome**

The polycystic ovarian syndrome (PCOS), and polycystic ovary morphology, both manifestations of insulin resistance, are very common in Type 1 women, and may be more common in intensively treated patients, and those with high insulin doses (Codner et al. 2006). Both PCOS (Rotterdam criteria) and biochemical hyperandrogenism occur in 40% to 50% of Type 1 women in their 20s (compared with a background prevalence in non-diabetic individuals of 5% to 10%), oligomenorrhoea in 20%, and hirsutism (which may be less of a clinical problem in diabetic compared with non-diabetic women) in about

30%. The ovarian androgen origin is confirmed by the absence of increase in LH and LH:FSH ratio in Type 1 patients (compared with the primary adrenal origin in non-diabetic individuals). Adjuvant metformin treatment (see Chapter 4) could be considered in women presenting with predominant oligomenorrhoea, or PCOS-associated infertility.

References

Cholesterol Treatment Trialists' (CTT) Collaborators; Kearney PM, Blackwell L, Collins R *et al.* (2008). Efficacy of cholesterol-lowering therapy in 18,686 people with diabetes in 14 randomised trials of statins: a meta-analysis. *Lancet*, **371**: 117–25. [PMID: 18191683]

Cleary PA, Orchard TJ, Genuth S *et al.*; Diabetes Control and Complications Trial/Epidemiology of Diabetes Interventions and Complications (DDCT/EDIC) Research Group (2006). The effect of intensive glycemic treatment on coronary artery calcification in type 1 participants of the Diabetes Control and Complications Trial/Epidemiology of Diabetes Interventions and Complications (DCCT/EDIC) Study. *Diabetes*, **55**: 3556–65. [PMID: 17130504]

Codner E, Soto N, Lopez P *et al.* (2006). Diagnostic criteria for polycystic ovary syndrome and ovarian morphology in women with hirsutism in type 1 diabetes mellitus. *J Clin Endocrinol Metab*, **91**: 2250–6. [PMID: 16569737]

Diabetes Control and Complications Trial Research Group (1995). Implementation of treatment protocols in the Diabetes Control and Complications Trial. *Diabetes Care*, **18**: 361–76. [PMID: 7555480]

Hurks R, Eisinger MJ, Goovaerts I *et al.* (2009). Early endothelial dysfunction in young type 1 diabetics. *Eur J Endovasc Surg*, **37**: 611–5. [PMID: 19297215]

Jenkins AJ, Lyons TJ, Zheng D *et al.*; the DCCT/EDIC Research Group (2003). Serum lipoproteins in the Diabetes Control and Complications Trial/Epidemiology of Diabetes Intervention and Complications cohort. *Diabetes Care*, **26**: 810–8. [PMID: 12610042]

Juutilainen A, Lehto S, Rönemaa T, Pyörälä K, Laakso M (2008). Similarity of the impact of type 1 and type 2 diabetes on cardiovascular mortality in middle-aged subjects. *Diabetes Care*, **31**: 714–9. [PMID: 18083789]

Laing SP, Swerdlow AJ, Carpenter LM *et al.* (2003). Mortality from cerebrovascular disease in a cohort of 23,000 patients with insulin-treated diabetes. *Stroke*, **34**: 418–21. [PMID: 12574553]

Laing SP, Swerdlow AJ, Slater SD *et al.* (1999). The British Diabetic Association Cohort Study: 1. All-cause mortality in patients with insulin-treated diabetes mellitus. *Diabet Med*, **16**: 459–65. [PMID: 10391392]

Larsen K, Brekke M, Sandvik L, Arnesen H, Hanssen KF, Dahl-Jørgensen K (2002). Silent coronary atheromatosis in type 1 diabetic patients and its relation to long-term glycemic control. *Diabetes*, **51**: 2637–41. [PMID: 12145181]

Levy DM, Galton D (2005). Diabetes, lipids, and atherosclerosis. Chapter 135 in: *Endocrinology*, 5th edn. De Groot LJ, Jameson JL (eds). Elsevier. ISBN: 978–0–72–160376–6

Molitch ME (2006). Management of dyslipidemias in patients with diabetes and chronic kidney disease. *Clin J Am Soc Nephrol*, **1**: 1090–9. [PMID: 17699330]

Nathan DM, Cleary PA, Backlund JY et al.; Diabetes Control and Complications Trial/Epidemiology of Diabetes Interventions and Complications (DCCT/EDIC) Study Research Group (2005). Intensive diabetes treatment and cardiovascular disease in patients with type 1 diabetes. *N Engl J Med*, **353**: 2643–53. [PMID: 16371630]

Nathan DM, Lachin J, Cleary P et al.; The Diabetes Control and Complications Trial/Epidemiology of Diabetes Interventions and Complications Research Group (2003). Intensive diabetes therapy and carotid intima–media thickness in type 1 diabetes mellitus. *N Engl J Med*, **348**: 2294–303. [PMID: 12788993]

Pambianco G, Costacou T, Orchard TJ (2007). The prediction of major outcomes of Type 1 diabetes: a 12-year prospective evaluation of three separate definitions of the metabolic syndrome and their components and estimated glucose disposal rate: the Pittsburgh Epidemiology of Diabetes Complications Study experience. *Diabetes Care*, **30**: 1248–54. [PMID: 17303788]

Rabago Rodriguez R, Gomez-Diaz RA, Tanhus Haj J et al. (2007). Carotid intima–media thickness in pediatric type 1 diabetes patients. *Diabetes Care*, **30**: 2599–602. [PMID: 17644614]

Stehouwer CD, Henry RMA, Ferreira I (2008). Arterial stiffness and the metabolic syndrome: a pathway to cardiovascular disease. *Diabetologia*, **51**: 527–39. [PMID: 18239908]

Zgibor JC, Platt GA, Ruppert K, Orchard TJ, Roberts MS (2006). Deficiencies of cardiovascular risk prediction models for type 1 diabetes. *Diabetes Care*, **29**: 1860–5. [PMID: 16873793]

Further reading

Fisher BM (2002). *Heart Disease and Diabetes (Advances in Diabetes)*. Informa Healthcare. ISBN: 978–1–84–184220–2

Fisher M (ed) (2008). *Heart Disease and Diabetes (Oxford Diabetes Library)*. Oxford University Press. ISBN: 978–0–19–954372–4

Pignone M, Alberts MJ, Colwell JA et al.; American Diabetes Association; American Heart Association; American College of Cardiology Foundation. Aspirin for primary prevention of cardiovascular events in people with diabetes: a position statement of the American Diabetes Association, a scientific statement of the American Heart Association, and an expert consensus document of the American College of Cardiology Foundation (2010). *Diabetes Care*, **33**: 1395–402. [PMID: 20508233]

Chapter 7

Adolescence and emerging adulthood

Key points

- During puberty and adolescence there are profound changes in endocrinology, especially in the growth hormone axis, but their contribution to vascular complications is still not clear.
- Microvascular complications occur from puberty onwards. The contribution of prepubertal duration to microvascular complications is less than that of pubertal duration, but is not negligible.
- Advanced microvascular complications are probably less prevalent now than in the past, though there is little systematic evidence that glycaemic control has improved in this age group.
- Hypertension, especially systolic, is frequent, and is probably related to multifactorial premature arterial stiffness. Subtle changes in lipid profile may contribute, but their impact is not known. Cigarette smoking is still common, probably underestimated, and clinical teams need to do more to improve cessation rates.
- The evidence base for treatment of identified macrovascular risk factors is weak, and only a small proportion is currently treated pharmacologically.
- Transition to adult care is difficult, should be managed actively, and must take into account the high prevalence of psychosocial morbidity in subgroups, especially young women with eating disorders.

7.1 Introduction

Puberty is a critical time in Type 1 diabetes, during which a combination of rapidly changing physiology, especially increasing insulin resistance, and behavioural changes pose a combined challenge to glycaemic control, which nearly always deteriorates, and generally remains poor until late adolescence, though most studies find that glycaemia improves in young people from their late teens and early 20s onwards. This important stage is usually termed 'young adulthood' but the full adult personality does not emerge until the late 20s; the variable intervening time (shorter in lower socioeconomic groups and in rural compared with urban individuals) is probably best termed 'emerging adulthood' (Weissberg-Benchell *et al.* 2007). During this period individuals are fluid geographically (including the important and poorly studied university period), emotionally, and economically. This whole period, but particularly early adolescence, may set the stage for accelerated microvascular complications, particularly in a subgroup of females with persistent behavioural problems (especially diet, and insulin manipulation and omission to reduce weight) and overt mental health problems, often associated with disastrous glycaemic control. The aims of diabetes care in adolescence are therefore to optimize glycaemic control in order to reduce the risk of long-term complications, to maintain normal physical and psychosocial development, and to give support to the young person and their family to help them develop strategies to cope with a potentially very long duration of an unstable chronic condition.

7.2 Changes in endocrinology

Insulin resistance and body fat increase early, between Tanner stage 1 (prepuberty) and stage 2, the earliest detectable clinical stage of puberty. The contribution of gonadal steroids to insulin resistance is not clear: levels are even higher in adults than adolescents, at a time when insulin sensitivity starts improving again.

Deterioration in glycaemic control is almost inevitable during puberty. Emerging behavioural, psychological, and psychosocial problems contribute to different degrees in individuals (see Chapter 8) but abnormalities in the GH–IGF-1 axis are the most important physiological factors. Portal insulin deficiency decreases hepatic production of IGF-I and its major binding protein IGFBP-3, but increases IGFBP-1 which is a major negative regulator of IGF-1 (Figure 7.1). IGF-1, acting through its receptor, has direct insulin-like effects at the liver and in the periphery, increasing glucose metabolism via insulin-independent mechanisms; in addition low IGF-I levels results in the linear growth failure that was previously so common in Type 1 diabetes but which is almost never seen nowadays, presumably because of improved insulin treatment. Decreased hypothalamic–pituitary feedback inhibition of GH secretion leads to higher basal GH levels, GH pulse frequency and amplitudes, which mediate the metabolic effects of insulin resistance (increased hepatic glucose production and lipolysis, and decreased insulin-mediated muscle glucose uptake). The clinical importance of this mechanism is supported by the beneficial

Figure 7.1 The GH–IGF-1 axis in Type 1 diabetes and its role in increasing insulin resistance

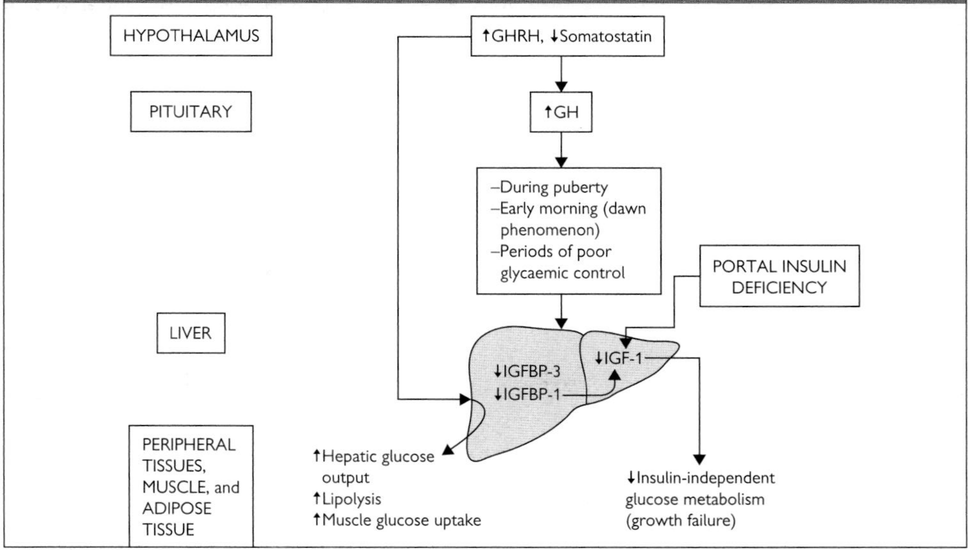

HYPOTHALAMUS

↑GHRH, ↓Somatostatin

PITUITARY

↑GH

–During puberty
–Early morning (dawn phenomenon)
–Periods of poor glycaemic control

PORTAL INSULIN DEFICIENCY

↓IGF-1

↓IGFBP-3
↓IGFBP-1

↓Insulin-independent glucose metabolism (growth failure)

LIVER

PERIPHERAL TISSUES, MUSCLE, and ADIPOSE TISSUE

↑Hepatic glucose output
↑Lipolysis
↑Muscle glucose uptake

CHAPTER 7 **Adolescence & emerging adulthood**

effects of recombinant IGF-1/IGFBP-3 on insulin requirements and insulin sensitivity in a clinical trial in adolescents and young adults, associated with significantly lower overnight GH levels (Saukkonen *et al.* 2004).

7.2.1 Endocrine abnormalities and diabetic complications

Experimental studies link growth hormone (GH) and insulin-like growth factor I (IGF-I) with complications, but the clinical evidence is inconsistent. The classical observations are that hypopituitary patients do not develop diabetic retinopathy, and that hypophysectomy can improve retinopathy, but conversely acromegalic patients with diabetes do not have an increased risk of retinopathy. Somatostatin analogues and other GH antagonist treatments are being investigated in diabetic retinopathy, but these drugs may act only partly via the GH axis—direct anti-angiogenic and anti-apoptotic effects may also be important. GH and IGF-I are unlikely to play a role in renal complications, though there is a lot of experimental evidence implicating them. Likewise, there is no clear link between sex steroids and microvascular complications.

7.3 Duration of prepubertal Type 1 diabetes and its contribution to microvascular complications

There has been much research in this area. The consensus is that prepubertal Type 1 diabetes, while not conferring protection against subsequent development of microvascular complications, contributes less than postpubertal duration. A Swedish survey found that diabetes onset before the age of 10 yrs is associated with a much lower rate of progression to diabetic nephropathy than with onset between 10 and 14 yrs. There were no cases of ESRD in those diagnosed under the age of 5. This very early onset group seems to be particularly protected against renal and retinal complications, for reasons that are not known: the time to developing complications was increased by ~3 yrs in a study in young Australians—though glycaemic control exerts a powerful and independent effect (Donaghue *et al.* 2003). While the relative protective effect of very early onset should not be used as a reason not to attempt to establish good control early on, it does leave welcome room for manoeuvre in these very young people where their parents' major concern is hypoglycaemia.

Regardless of glycaemic control, microvascular complications are rare before puberty. Puberty, however, accelerates the development of microvascular complications, both microalbuminuria and retinopathy, with a three- to fourfold increased risk. Therefore, while the onset of complications is delayed in those with prepubertal onset, the Berlin Retinopathy Study and the Oxford Regional Study both found that retinopathy progression is more rapid in children with prepubertal compared with pubertal onset of diabetes. Retinopathy may progress very rapidly after the onset of puberty, and there have been occasional reports of pre-proliferative changes in pubertal 11-yr olds (Schultz et al. 2002).

7.4 Glycaemic control in adolescents and young adults

7.4.1 Diabetes Control and Complications Trial (DCCT)/Epidemiology of Diabetes Interventions and Complications (EDIC)

There were 195 adolescents (13 to 17 yrs old at study entry) in the DCCT, with a mean age of 15 yrs, and with a mean baseline A1C between 9.3% and 10.1%. During DCCT the mean A1C in both groups was higher than in the whole DCCT cohort (conventional 9.8%, intensive 8.1%). A1C levels converged within the first 4 yrs of EDIC after DCCT close-out, much as in the whole study group, though again at a slightly higher level, 8.4% to 8.5%, compared with 8.1% to 8.2%. From the perspective of the beginning of the second decade of the 21st century, and nearly 20 yrs after DCCT ended, we are inclined to assume that there have been major improvements in glycaemia in this vulnerable group. Subsequent studies have largely disproved this comforting notion. Though not consistently so, A1C levels in adolescents even in recent cross-sectional studies are often very disappointing. Nearly 50% of adolescents in a UK study in 2002 had A1C >9%. Mean A1C in normoalbuminuric 18-yr olds in the Oxford Regional Study was 9.5%, and over 11% in those with intermittent or persistent microalbuminuria.

At follow-up at a mean age of 26 yrs, subjects who had entered the DCCT as adolescents had poorer control (mean A1C 8.4%) compared with those who had entered as adults (follow-up age of 36 yrs, mean A1C ~8.0%). Intensively treated adolescents were in worse control by the time they were young adults, a useful reminder that behavioural traits acquired as adolescents are not automatically correlated with good control as adults when subjected to the competing environmental and social demands of young adulthood. In the international Hvidøre Study, a continuing international survey, female adolescents aged 11 to 18 had significantly higher mean A1C than males (8.3% vs 8.1%) and those with language difficulties even higher levels (8.5%; de Beaufort et al. 2007).

7.4.2 Has glycaemic control improved in adolescents and young adults post-DCCT?

Views differ on whether or not there have been general improvements in glycaemic control in young people, especially in the post-DCCT period with its explosion of technological improvements, and increased emphasis on management and educational strategies. Individual centres have published encouraging and improving data, but reporting bias is inevitable, and some wider surveys are less positive (Box 7.1).

7.4.3 Insulin regimens and their relation to glycaemic control

The Hvidøre study provided a contemporary (2005) snapshot of insulin regimens in 2000 adolescents aged 11 to 18 yrs across 21 centres, mostly European (Figure 7.2). Mean A1C was 8.2%. Unexpectedly, twice-daily free-mixed regimens were associated with better glycaemic control (mean A1C 7.9%) than other regimens, including continuous subcutaneous insulin infusion (CSII), while twice-daily biphasic regimens carried the worst control (mean A1C 8.6%). However, control with any insulin regimen was good in those centres with overall low A1C levels. The regimen used is therefore less critical than the way in which it is implemented and the expertise—and experience—of the diabetes team. Perhaps the DCCT-inspired concept of 'intensive' control has carried a misleading message that multiple daily injections (MDI) or CSII *per se* will inevitably confer better glycaemic outcomes than more traditional regimens with which some teams may be comfortable and expert. This belief was undermined by the 2008 reanalysis of the DCCT data showing that for a given achieved A1C, 'intensive' treatment does *not* carry an improved microvascular outcome compared with 'conventional' treatment (Lachin *et al.* 2008; see Section 9.8.2). Characterizing traditional insulin regimens as 'old fashioned' or 'not modern' is unwise.

Box 7.1 Changes in glycaemic control over time in adolescents—international perspectives

- In the international Hvidøre Study between 1998 and 2005, there was no change in mean A1C (8.2%) in 11- to 18-yr olds across 21 centres (range 7.4% to 9.2%). The A1C ranking of the different centres also did not change. However, despite the wide differences in mean A1C, there were no differences between centres in rates of diabetic ketoacidosis (DKA) and severe hypoglycaemia
- Over a 12-yr period up to 2002, a major Australian centre also reported no change in median A1C (8.5%)
- Mean A1C remained unchanged at 9.2% in two cohorts of younger Scottish children under 15 studied in 1997–1998 and again in 2002–2004 (Scottish Study Group 2006)
- A continuing systematic countrywide survey from Germany has shown a slow but consistent fall in A1C in young people of mean age ~19 yrs, by about 0.06%/yr between 1995 and 2007

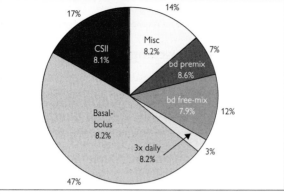

Figure 7.2 Snapshot of insulin regimens in young people (Hvidøre Study 2005). Proportions using regimens outside pie segments, mean A1C using those regimens inside segments

17%

CSII
8.1%

14%

Misc
8.2%

7%

bd premix
8.6%

12%

bd free-mix
7.9%

Basal-bolus
8.2%

3x daily
8.2%

3%

47%

7.4.4 CSII vs MDI

Meta-analysis in adults (see Section 4.5) suggests overall slightly improved glycaemic control with CSII compared with MDI. Inevitably, given the wide developmental range covered by the rubric 'children and adolescents', and the wide differences between centres in resourcing and experience in CSII, data are inconsistent and meta-analysis is hampered by the small number of analyzable trials. In addition, although A1C reduction is important, there are other outcomes of CSII that are less amenable to quantitative analysis, but nevertheless are of great, possibly primary, importance (this has been shown in several studies in pre-schoolers, where in comparison with MDI, glycaemia is unchanged, but treatment satisfaction, parental anxiety, and quality of life (QoL) show greater improvement). Undoubtedly where there is specific expertise and experience, results in adolescents (and children) can be remarkable, and CSII has been reported to reduce hospitalizations, emergency department visits, and DKA frequency even in adolescents with recurrent DKA, a group that at first sight would not conform to the ideal for CSII treatment. In addition, some studies have reported reluctance to stop pump treatment even when A1C deteriorated with treatment, confirming that CSII carries benefits for individuals that differ from their clinical teams' preoccupation with glycaemic control. A rigorous prospective comparison of CSII and MDI in a total of nearly 60 adolescents at the Steno Centre confirmed these subtle balances of pros and cons:

• A small, non-significant fall in A1C in both groups (CSII: −0.6%; MDI: −0.2%)

- Severe hypoglycaemia and insulin dose were slightly lower in the CSII group
- BMI increased, more in the CSII group
- DKA occurred only in the CSII group
- QoL scores and diet did not change (Johannesen *et al.* 2008).

7.5 Microvascular complications

7.5.1 Retinopathy

Screening for retinopathy in young people is contentious. The American Diabetes Association recommends annual retinopathy screening from the age of 10 yrs, and after longer duration than 3 to 5 yrs. A study in a major USA teaching centre detected virtually no retinopathy in groups of young people, apart from a small number of cases of transient minor background retinopathy up to the age of 22 yrs, but for an adolescent group they were in good glycaemic control, with mean A1C <8%. In contrast, hypertension and microalbuminuria were much more frequent than retinopathy, and it was suggested that retinopathy screening should be limited to patients with persistent high A1C, hypertension, or microalbuminuria (Huo *et al.* 2007). Even in more representative groups of young people, the current prevalence of retinopathy is low. Mild non-proliferative retinopathy was found in ~5% of a group of young French people (mean A1C 8.5%) attending a summer camp, and in the most recent of three sequential cross-sectional studies only 2% of an Australian group (mean age 15 yrs, duration 8 yrs) were found to have more than trivial retinopathy in both eyes, and this was not associated with higher A1C. The reduction in the prevalence of the same degree of retinopathy between 1990 and 2002 was dramatic (12% in the earliest cohort), yet median A1C had not changed (Mohsin *et al.* 2005).

Whichever screening protocol is adopted, clinically significant retinopathy in young people is thankfully now very uncommon, and minor retinopathy should be regarded primarily as a marker of poor glycaemic control, the presence of other complications, and the need for steps to be taken to improve control (see Section 5.3). However, since diabetes duration is such a powerful risk factor for retinopathy, adult (annual) screening protocols should be rigorously adopted from late teens onwards. Other diabetic eye complications are extremely rare in adolescence, though visually significant cataracts have been reported in patients as young as 12 yrs.

Intensive treatment in the adolescent DCCT cohort had the same beneficial effect as in the whole, adult, cohort—that is, risk reduction of about 60% for a three-step change in retinopathy, reflecting the similar differences between intensive and conventional groups, despite the higher absolute mean A1C in both groups.

There are large variations in the reported prevalence of standard definitions of microalbuminuria, and these are mostly accounted for by differences in duration and glycaemic control. In the large Oxford prospective cohort study the prevalence of microalbuminuria was 26% 10 yrs after diagnosis at a mean age of 9 yrs, increasing to 51% after 20 yrs (Amin *et al.* 2008). In contrast, the earliest cohort of Australians (1990) had a much lower prevalence, 7%, and an even lower prevalence, 3%, in the most recent cohort. Ten per cent of patients in another large UK cohort (mean age 14 yrs, duration only 6 yrs) had microalbuminuria (Moore and Shield 2000), and this suggests that higher levels of A1C are tolerated in the UK, with apparently deleterious effects on early microvascular complications. In the Oxford study, microalbuminuria first occurred at a median age of 16 yrs, and was more common in females. As in adults, more than 50% regressed to normoalbuminuria, but there was also a high relapse rate.

Macroalbuminuria occurred in 3% in the Oxford study, at a median age of 19 yrs and duration 10 yrs, again strongly predicted by glycaemia, but also by systolic blood pressure (BP). Smoking was not a risk factor in this and other studies, and overall it seems that smoking may be associated with the development of microalbuminuria, but not consistently with progression to macroalbuminuria. This uncertainty in no way, of course, detracts from the importance of smoking cessation in this age group (see below).

The screening strategy for microalbuminuria in young people is not agreed, but microalbuminuria is predicted by an acceleration in urinary albumin excretion rate from 11 yrs. Because albumin:creatinine ratios are highly variable, expert opinion is that it should be measured three times a year. The management strategy in young people with persistent microalbuminuria is even less clear. There is no RCT evidence for the benefit of ACE inhibitors in the under 18s, but persistent microalbuminuria in young people has a potentially more serious renal prognosis than in adult-onset Type 1 diabetes. After allowing a reasonable time to confirm that microalbuminuria is persistent and not transient, and optimizing glycaemic control (CSII could be a sound strategy in these circumstances), discuss starting ACE inhibitor treatment, with appropriate contraceptive precautions in females. As in adults, consider causes other than diabetes if significant microalbuminuria starts abruptly, there is clear hypertension, or abnormal urinalysis. A bold international long-term intervention study, proposed duration 4-5 yrs, using low-dose ACE inhibitor treatment (quinapril up to 10 mg daily) and atorvastatin 10 mg daily in a factorial double-blind trial (AdDIT) has recently started. Subjects aged between 11 and 16 yrs with microalbuminuria will be studied at the same time as a parallel non-interventional observational group. The primary outcome will be

AER, with secondary endpoints of other microvascular complications and intermediate measures of cardiovascular risk (e.g. carotid intimate-media thickness; AdDIT Research Group 2009).

In the DCCT, intensive treatment had no effect in preventing microalbuminuria—barely surprising in view of the small numbers—but microalbuminuria was significantly reduced in the secondary intervention group whose baseline mean albumin excretion rate was just at the threshold of microalbuminuria (26 to 29 mg/24 h). This is an important finding, and rigorous screening for microalbuminuria from mid-adolescence onwards is certainly warranted (DCCT Research Group 1994).

7.6 Macrovascular risk factors

Carotid intima–media thickness (CIMT), a surrogate non-invasive indicator of atherosclerosis in children and adolescents, is generally increased, though results are not always consistent, probably because reference ranges are narrow at this young age. Nevertheless, CIMT has generally been shown to be associated with age of onset of diabetes, systolic BP, and various lipid measurements, especially LDL. Systolic BP is probably the most important modifiable factor. Cross-sectional relationships between CIMT and A1C are inconsistent, though long-term prospective studies, for example the Oslo study confirm the expected association. Whether increased CIMT shortly after diagnosis in young people carries the same macrovascular risk as it does in adults is not clear, but it is an alert that there is early evidence of abnormal vasculature, even in the absence of overt risk factors.

7.6.1 Hypertension and lipids

7.6.1.1 Hypertension

BP increases with age in normal children. Most children with microalbuminuria are normotensive—but BP, especially systolic, in the high-normal range, may be important in the kidney which may already have abnormal autoregulation and blood flow. Genetic factors, including renin–angiotensin system insertion/deletion polymorphisms, may be significant, but widely different results have been found in cross-sectional studies. DCCT/EDIC found that the I/I ACE genotype was associated with a borderline lower risk for persistent microalbuminuria and nephropathy, but other polymorphisms may be more important, and so far there are no reliable genetic predictors of complications.

Hypertension is likely to be as important in adolescents with diabetes as it is in adults, but it is more difficult to diagnose, because gender, age, and height must be considered, and BP percentiles and not absolute thresholds should be used (>95th for hypertension, 90 to 95th for prehypertension). Normative data are available (National High

Blood Pressure Education Program Working Group 2004) and reference values for ambulatory BP measurements have also been published (Urbina *et al.* 2008). A large Norwegian study in young adolescents (mean age 13 yrs, duration 6 yrs) reported BP >95th percentile in the expected 4% of cases, though persistent microalbuminuria was present in only 1%, suggesting that 'essential' hypertension is common in young Type 1 patients (Margeirsdottir *et al.* 2008). This is confirmed in an older Finnish population, including those aged 20 upwards (Rönnback *et al.* 2004). Age-related changes in BP were similar to non-diabetic people, but occurred 15 to 20 yrs earlier. These included consistently higher systolic BP at all ages, and diastolic BP that starts to decline earlier than in non-diabetic people, yielding a strikingly higher pulse pressure at all ages and durations of diabetes, indicating accelerated arterial ageing and stiffening. The prevalence of hypertension (BP ≥140/≥90) was ~15% in the 18 to 24 yrs age group, increasing to ~20% to 25% in those aged 25 to 40. By age 30 to 34 yrs, pulse pressure was higher than controls at all levels of albuminuria and increased with the degree of albuminuria. Practitioners should be actively seeking evidence of hypertension, even in the absence of microalbuminuria, from mid-teens onwards, regardless of the age of diagnosis. USA guidelines for the management of hypertension are shown in Box 7.2.

7.6.1.2 *Lipids*

Conventional lipid profiles are generally indistinguishable from (or in some studies better than) non-diabetic contemporaries. However the Norwegian study found LDL cholesterol above ADA recommended levels (>2.6 mmol/L) in 35% of their young cohort, and 7% had low HDL cholesterol (<1.1 mmol/L). The recommendation is to consider lipid-lowering medication when LDL ≥4.1 mmol/L (or ≥3.4 mmol/L in those at high cardiovascular risk). However, there is no evidence base for early primary intervention with medication, and in practice long-term lipid-lowering treatment in young people under 18 yrs, and even in the young adult group, is very uncommon. High dietary fat and low fibre intake were common in the Norwegians, and no doubt in many other countries, and intensive dietary input is probably a more practicable approach. Non-pharmacological intervention with nutraceutical products such as plant stanols may be effective and more acceptable for modest LDL elevations in this group. Aspirin is contraindicated in those under 21, and there is no evidence for its benefit in young adults.

Box 7.2 Management of hypertension in children and adolescents

- Prehypertension (90 to 95th percentile): lifestyle intervention for 3 to 6 months, recommending increased physical activity, weight control, and dietary intervention (salt restriction, increase in fresh fruit, vegetables, and fibre—similar to the evidence-based dietary approaches to stop hypertension (DASH) diet in adults): www.nhlbi.nih.gov/health/public/heart/hbp/dash/new_dash.pdf
- Consider pharmacological treatment if after 3 to 6 months BP remains >95th percentile (or >130/80 if 95th percentile is higher than this)
- First-line treatment is a once-daily ACE inhibitor (e.g. lisinopril, fosinopril, quinapril) or ARB (e.g. losartan) if side effects

7.6.2 Smoking

Regular smoking in non-diabetic children and adolescents is associated with a 50% to 75% increased risk of cardiovascular events in later life, and tobacco use was associated with progression of retinopathy in the DCCT. Only 3% of the Norwegians 12 yrs or older with diabetes admitted to smoking, but occasional tobacco use is much more frequent in other studies—up to 35% of white 10- to 20-yr olds were ever-smokers, and nearly 30% had smoked within the past year in one study. Almost 50% had detectable urinary cotinine in another study where the median age of starting smoking was 16 yrs. In EDIC subjects in their early 40s, with more than 20 yrs duration, 14% to 18% were still smoking. The vast majority of smokers are aware of the harmful effects on general health and on specific diabetic complications (Tyc and Throckmorton-Belzer 2006). Systematic questioning of young people about tobacco use from mid-teens onwards, and access to smoking cessation programmes is important, though probably neglected in most clinics. In addition, discussing subjects such as smoking (and alcohol, and contraception) is often difficult when parents are present, and unaware of the personal habits of their children, especially if they are under the legal age for these activities.

7.6.3 Exercise

The beneficial metabolic effects of exercise in Type 1 patients are clear, particularly where there are added insulin resistance characteristics. Clinical studies have shown less consistent beneficial effects, partly because their focus is usually short-term glycaemic control and management of hypoglycaemia during exercise and not long-term cardiovascular risk factors. However, in a large study of 3- to 18-yr olds in Germany, regular physical activity three or more times a week was associated with a significantly lower A1C (mean ~0.3% lower) in all age groups, and with less dyslipidaemia (total cholesterol, triglycerides, and HDL) in older adolescents (15 to 18 yrs). Prevalence of diastolic, but not systolic, hypertension, was lower in those doing more exercise. In view of the certain benefits of regular exercise, it is striking that 45% of these young people were physically inactive (Herbst *et al.* 2007).

7.7 The emergence of advanced diabetic complications in young adulthood

In contrast with adolescence, where advanced tissue complications are rarely seen, the picture changes in transition to young adulthood where the combination of lengthening duration, poor control, and adverse psychosocial factors conspires to paint a more concerning picture.

By the time patients reach their early 20s, increased mortality can already be detected. In contrast with earlier studies from the 1980s, where much of the excess mortality was due to renal disease, the Diabetes UK/British Diabetic Association study of Type 1 people under 40 (Laing *et al.* 2005) found that deaths from acute causes was much more common than those resulting from long-term complications; acute deaths in turn were strongly associated with living alone, past drug abuse, and those needing psychiatric referral. There was no relation between these factors and death from chronic complications, which however was associated with poor socio-economic status (and the expected hypertension, renal disease, and neuropathy).

An extensive study in Oxford has looked in detail at physical, psychological, and psychosocial morbidity associated with Type 1 diabetes. Young adults were studied at mean age 22 yrs, duration 10 yrs, and again 10 yrs later in their mid-30s (Bryden *et al.* 2003). Glycaemic control remained constant, with A1C levels between 8% and 9% over the whole period, slightly worse in women, but with this much longer duration 20% to 30% had required laser treatment for retinopathy, and 2% each dialysis and toe amputation. Major complications were about three times more frequent in women. Serious psychiatric illness requiring hospital assessment occurred in 18%, much higher than in the background population, and was associated with recurrent DKA. Fourteen percent of women had attempted or committed suicide, and two had died of diabetic renal disease. The microvascular complication rate was similar to that in the EURODIAB complications study, but the extent and severity of the adverse psychiatric outcomes emphasizes the importance of identifying the most at-risk young adults, and ensuring that medical, psychological, and psychiatric support are adequate in this group (see Chapter 8).

7.8 'Brittle' diabetes

Unstable glycaemic control unresponsive to intensive management, including attempts at CSII, and usually occurring in young women, has been described as 'brittle diabetes'. The literature on this contentious and fortunately uncommon condition comes largely from the UK and USA. It may form a discrete syndrome, characterized by onset at puberty, recurrent hospital admissions (some patients have predominant hypoglycaemia, others predominant DKA), overweight, high insulin requirements, long-term oligo/amenorrhoea, and major psychosocial disruption (Saunders and Williams 2004). Eating disorders, gastroparesis, and serious disruption of family dynamics are frequent accompaniments. 'Brittle diabetes' also occurs in males, but much less frequently, and there is an analogous condition in the elderly (see Chapter 9), where however psychosocial factors seem to be less prominent than in the younger patients. Despite the apparent insulin resistance and high insulin requirements, in the small numbers of patients fitted with implantable insulin pumps, actual insulin requirements are not exceptional. Insulin omission is therefore likely, and extreme examples of treatment manipulation have been documented. The few follow-up studies have documented high levels of microvascular complications, poor pregnancy outcomes, and possibly of death. For patients, their families, and their diabetes teams, this is one of the most taxing and stressful clinical situations in Type 1 diabetes. There is no agreement on the best approach, and an individualized programme of medical, educational, and behavioural therapies should be planned and agreed. The degree of brittleness fluctuates with the level of psychosocial stresses, but fortunately seems to improve with time, and it is rare beyond the age of 30.

7.9 Hypoglycaemia and neurocognitive function

Severe hypoglycaemia (assistance, coma, and seizure) in the intensive DCCT group was much higher than in the adult cohort, despite the shorter duration and higher overall A1C levels, probably due to the higher insulin doses, and the more erratic exercise and eating habits of adolescents compared with adults. However, neurocognitive function in the EDIC follow-up was not significantly impaired in the intensive group, despite the higher hypoglycaemia rate, and should encourage both screening for early complications in this group, and intensification of treatment wherever possible (Musen *et al.* 2008). These surprisingly good neurocognitive outcomes are strikingly different from those with childhood onset of diabetes.

7.10 Transition to the adult diabetes service

This is a topic of major importance and has not been given the prominence it deserves. The second decade of Type 1 diabetes usually coincides with the period between late adolescence and early adulthood. Early complications may be developing, though established complications are uncommon. Many late adolescents are in poor glycaemic control, and it is a critical period for the diabetes team to engage with the young people to optimize control. Most post-adolescents with Type 1 diabetes continue normal psychosocial development, but they have specific needs, highlighted by the Oxford study, especially young women with eating disorders. In addition, this group needs specific attention to manageable factors that may lead to continuing poor self-care, for example alcohol and drug abuse, and mental illness. They also need careful screening for microvascular complications, and sensitive assessment for angiotensin blockade, antihypertensive, and statin treatment, tailored with an individualized approach to discussion of long-term complications and their implications.

7.10.1 University

This is a long and important period for young people, usually 3 yrs, but is often viewed as a holding period during which active management of diabetes does not occur. Although students will register with their university primary health-care services, most will not have access to specialist services during term-time, and many will attend their home hospital diabetes service during vacations, amounting therefore perhaps to only three consultations a year. Access arrangements for specialist services vary in different countries. For example in Denmark diabetes care is transferred to the local teaching hospital during the students' university stay, an arrangement that may help stabilize or even improve glycaemia during this period. A study in the UK found that although glycaemic control did not improve at university, interestingly weight did not change either, suggesting a degree of frugality of the student diet, increased activity, or both (Geddes *et al.* 2006). The home diabetes team should proactively discuss relevant and important matters with the students, including alcohol, diet (which often abruptly changes in frequency, quality, and quantity once parental influences on feeding habits have waned), sexual health, including contraception, reinforcement of the sick-day rules, and liaising with the university health service about medical histories and prescription requirements.

7.10.2 Transition to adult care

Conventionally run adult outpatient diabetes clinics are a poor environment in which to hold detailed discussions of the specific problems associated with young adulthood; however, simply instituting a clinic for young adults, not surprisingly, does not ensure improved control after transfer from a paediatric clinic. For example, only those in the highest tertile of A1C benefited from a young adult clinic compared with a general endocrine clinic in young Americans aged 15 to 25 yrs. All others remained with A1C levels between 8.4% and 9.0%, apart from those on CSII, who consistently achieved A1C levels 1% lower at all ages (Lane et al. 2007).

Centres whose patients significantly improved their glycaemic control have often achieved this through a fundamental rethink of their whole service provision, for example increased numbers of visits and diabetes specialist nurses, frequent staff meetings, and written patient information. Specific initiatives used in Manitoba, Canada, in a transition service for 18- to 30-yr olds included a 'health navigator', an administrative co-ordinator facilitating email and telephone communication between the young adults and the various components of the adult diabetes service, and multiple interaction channels, including a website, newsletter, informal drop-in events, and patient discussion and support groups (Weissberg-Benchell et al. 2007). Even this level of organizational input is not guaranteed to improve metabolic control, but discussion, reassurance, and good communication can ease the transition from a paediatric care environment that may have been comforting and stable for more than 10 yrs. Young people see the adult clinic as formal and not really in tune with their needs, and the presence of a paediatrician in the transition clinic provides reassurance of continuity of care.

Studies have identified multiple factors that probably contribute to improved care of the young adult with Type 1 diabetes. While evident, and widely acknowledged to be self-evident, there are few examples of exemplary practice in the area, and insufficient studies of outcomes (Box 7.3).

> **Box 7.3 Factors facilitating transition from paediatric to adult diabetes services (adapted from Weissberg-Benchell et al. 2007)**
>
> - Getting adequate information about transition
> - Maintaining the informality of the paediatric clinic approach while increasing vigilance for emerging microvascular complications, especially early microalbuminuria and retinopathy
> - Continuity of care by clinicians—presence of both paediatric and adult physicians
> - Ensuring rapid follow-up once discharged from the paediatric/adolescent clinic—delays, often more than 6 months, probably lead to default
> - Address concerns expressed by paediatricians (and patients and their families) about quality of care in the adult service
> - Specific training for physicians who deal only with adults on the needs of young adults and their specific problems, for example eating disorders, alcohol and drug problems, mental health problems, sexual health and contraception
> - Instituting administrative (e.g. transition co-ordinator) or clinical personnel (e.g. diabetes educator/specialist nurse with an interest in adolescent diabetes) to aid transition
> - Written transition plans

References

Adolescent type 1 Diabetes Cardio-renal Intervention Trial Research Group (2009). Adolescent type 1 Diabetes Cardio-renal Intervention Trial (AdDIF). *BMC Paediatr*, **9**: 79. [PMID: 20017932]

Amin R, Widmer B, Prevost AT et al. (2008). Risk of microalbuminuria and progression to macroalbuminuria in a cohort with childhood onset type 1 diabetes: prospective observational study. *BMJ*, **336**: 697–701. [PMID: 18349042]

de Beaufort CE, Swift PG, Skinner CT et al.; Hvidoere Study Group on Childhood Diabetes 2005 (2007). Continuing stability of center differences in pediatric diabetes care: do advances in diabetes treatment improve outcome? The Hvidoere Study Group on Childhood Diabetes. *Diabetes Care*, **30**: 2245–50. [PMID: 17540955]

Bryden KS, Dunger DB, Mayou RA, Peveler RC, Neil HA (2003). Poor prognosis of young adults with type 1 diabetes: a longitudinal study. *Diabetes Care*, **26**: 1052–7. [PMID: 12663572]

Donaghue KC, Fairchild JM, Craig ME et al. (2003). Do all prepubertal years of diabetes duration contribute equally to diabetes complications? *Diabetes Care*, **26**: 1224–9. [PMID: 12663601]

Diabetes Control and Complications Research Group (1994). Effect of intensive diabetes treatment on the development and progression of long-term complications in adolescents with insulin-dependent diabetes mellitus: Diabetes Control and Complications Trial. *J Pediatr*, **125**: 177–88. [PMID: 8040759]

Geddes J, McGeough E, Frier BM (2006). Young adults with Type 1 diabetes in tertiary education: do students receive adequate specialist care? *Diabet Med*, **23**: 1155–7. [PMID: 16978384]

Herbst A, Kordonouri O, Schwab KO, Schmidt F, Holl RW (2007). Impact of physical activity on cardiovascular risk factors in children with type 1 diabetes: a multicenter study of 23,251 patients. *Diabetes Care*, **30**: 2098–100. [PMID: 17468347]

Huo B, Steffen AT, Swan K, Sikes K, Weinzimer SA, Tamborlane WV (2007). Clinical outcomes and cost-effectiveness of retinopathy screening in youth with type 1 diabetes. *Diabetes Care*, **30**: 362–3. [PMID: 17259509]

Johannesen J, Eising S, Kohlwes S et al. (2008). Treatment of Danish adolescent diabetic patients with CSII—a matched study to MDI. *Pediatr Diabetes*, **9**: 23–8. [PMID: 18211633]

Lachin JM, Genuth S, Nathan DM, Zinman B, Rutledge BN; DCCT/EDIC Research Group (2008). Effect of glycemic exposure on the risk of microvascular complications in the Diabetes Control and Complications Trial—revisited. *Diabetes*, **57**: 995–1001. [PMID: 18223010]

Laing SP, Jones ME, Swerdlow AJ, Burden AC, Gatling W (2005). Psychosocial and socioeconomic risk factors for premature death in young people with type 1 diabetes. *Diabetes Care*, **28**: 1618–23. [PMID: 15983310]

Lane JT, Ferguson A, Hall J et al. (2007). Glycemic control over 3 years in a young adult clinic for patients with type 1 diabetes. *Diabetes Res Clin Pract*, **78**: 385–91. [PMID: 17602780]

Margeirsdottir HD, Larsen JR, Brunborg C, Overby NC, Dahl-Jørgensen K; Norwegian Study Group for Childhood Diabetes (2008). High prevalence of cardiovascular risk factors in children and adolescents with type 1 diabetes: a population-based study. *Diabetologia*, **51**: 554–61. [PMID: 18196217]

Mohsin F, Craig ME, Cusumano J et al. (2005). Discordant trends in microvascular complications in adolescents with type 1 diabetes from 1990 to 2002. *Diabetes Care*, **28**: 1974–80. [PMID: 16043741]

Moore TH, Shield JP; Microalbuminuria in diabetic adolescents and children (MIDAC) research group (2000). Prevalence of abnormal urinary albumin excretion in adolescents and children with insulin dependent diabetes: the MIDAC study. *Arch Dis Child*, **83**: 239–43. [PMID: 10952644]

Musen G, Jacobson AM, Ryan CM et al.; DCCT/EDIC Research Group (2008). The impact of diabetes and its treatment on cognitive function among adolescents who participated in the DCCT. *Diabetes Care*, **31**: 1933–8. [PMID: 18606979]

Rönnback M, Fagerudd J, Forsblom C et al.; Finnish Diabetic Nephropathy (FinnDiane) Study Group (2004). Altered age-related blood pressure pattern in type 1 diabetes. *Circulation*, **110**: 1076–82. [PMID: 15326070]

Saukkonen T, Amin R, Williams RM et al. (2004). Dose-dependent effects of recombinant human insulin-like growth factor (IGF)-1/IGF binding protein-3 complex on overnight growth hormone secretion and insulin sensitivity in type 1 diabetes. *J Clin Endocrinol Metab*, **89**: 4634–41. [PMID: 15356074]

Saunders SA, Williams G (2004). Difficult diabetes. Chapter 87 in: *International Textbook of Diabetes Mellitus*, 3rd edn. DeFronzo, Ferrannini, Keen, Zimmet (eds). Wiley. ISBN: 978–0–47–148655–8

Schultz CJ, Amin R, Dunger DB (2002). Markers of microvascular complications in insulin dependent diabetes. *Arch Dis Child*, **87**: 10–2. [PMID: 12089111]

Scottish Study Group for the care of the young with diabetes (2006). A longitudinal observational study of insulin therapy and glycaemic control in Scottish children with Type 1 diabetes: DIABAUD 3. *Diabet Med*, **23**: 1216–21. [PMID: 17054598]

Tyc VL, Throckmorton-Belzer L (2006). Smoking rates and the state of smoking interventions for children and adolescents with chronic illness. *Pediatrics*, **118**: e471–87. [PMID: 16882787]

Weissberg-Benchell J, Wolpert H, Anderson BJ (2007). Transitioning from pediatric to adult care: a new approach to the post-adolescent young person with type 1 diabetes. *Diabetes Care*, **30**: 2441–6. [PMID: 17666466]

Further reading

American Diabetes Association (2003). Management of dyslipidemia in children and adolescents with diabetes. *Diabetes Care*, **26**: 2194–7. [PMID: 12832334]

DASH (Dietary Approaches to Stop Hypertension). www.nhlbi.nih.gov/health/public/heart/hbp/dash/new_dash.pdf (site accessed 25.07.10).

Haire-Joshu D, Glasgow RE, Tibbs TL; American Diabetes Association (2004). Smoking and diabetes. *Diabetes Care*, **27** (Suppl 1): S74–5. [PMID: 14693932]

Hanas R (2006). *Type 1 Diabetes in Children, Adolescents and Young Adults*, 3rd revised edn. Class Publishing. ISBN: 978–1–859591–75–8

National High Blood Pressure Education Program Working Group on High Blood Pressure in Children and Adolescents (2004). The fourth report on the diagnosis, evaluation, and treatment of high blood pressure in children and adolescents. *Pediatrics*, **114** (2 Suppl 4th Report): 555–76. [PMID: 15286277]

Urbina E, Alpert B, Flynn J et al.; American Heart Association Atherosclerosis, Hypertension, and Obesity in Youth Committee (2008). Ambulatory blood pressure monitoring in children and adolescents: recommendations for standard assessment: a scientific statement from the American Heart Association Atherosclerosis, Hypertension, and Obesity in Youth Committee of the council on cardiovascular disease in the young and the council for high blood pressure research. *Hypertension*, **52**: 433–51. [PMID: 18678786]

132

Chapter 8

Psychological problems

Key points

- Psychological disturbances are common at all stages of diabetes, from diagnosis to the experience of late tissue complications.

- The most profound disturbances occur in young females, from early adolescence onwards, often manifested as a range of eating disorders associated with manipulation of insulin dosing.

- Quality of life broadly improves with better glycaemic control in the real-life setting.

- Depression is common, often not diagnosed, and frequently relapses. It should be actively sought out.

- The causes of family dysfunction, which is common, are multiple, but usually centre around issues of blood glucose control. Family dysfunction is associated with recurrent diabetic ketoacidosis. Cognitive behaviour therapy is effective, particularly in young people.

- Less intensive interventions designed to guide change in the absence of overt psychological difficulties, such as motivational interviewing, also seem to be valuable in young people.

8.1 Introduction

That there is an intimate relationship between diabetes, as with any other long-term illness, and psychological function and dysfunction, is evident. However, diabetes is unique among the chronic illnesses in its absence of signs, to their family, friends, colleagues—and to the people themselves who have diabetes, with the obvious exception of symptoms relating to hypo- or hyperglycaemia. This is particularly the case in the first 10 to 20 yrs of diabetes, when any evidence of tissue complications is usually barely apparent. The manifestations of psychological and psychosocial stress are therefore often subtle, frequently ignored, usually not managed or treated, and inevitably have an impact, severe in some, on the biomarkers of glycaemic control and their tissue counterparts. The Diabetes Control and Complications Trial (DCCT), with its emphasis on intensified management at all ages, has highlighted the family and social stresses suffered by many people with Type 1 diabetes. Some of these have already been discussed in relation to young people (Chapter 7). This chapter will highlight some of the recent progress in the diagnosis and management of psychological problems at different stages of Type 1 diabetes.

8.2 Diagnosis and immediate aftermath

Initial psychological reactions to the diagnosis are similar to those in other chronic conditions, namely sadness, anxiety, withdrawal, and dependence. Around one-third of children develop a clinical adjustment disorder in the period 3 to 12 months after diagnosis; although this usually resolves, persistence predicts later psychological difficulties (Cameron et al. 2007). Incidence rates of major depression, conduct, and generalized anxiety disorders were at their highest in the first year after diagnosis. These are associated with high rates of post-traumatic stress disorder in parents a year after diagnosis—up to 20% in mothers and 8% in fathers.

There have been a few studies, necessarily retrospective, of psychosocial function in Type 1 patients and their families in the period before diagnosis. A large Swedish case–control study found that other than a hint of increased isolation, if anything there were fewer stressful events in this period. However, hospitalization or serious illness was more likely than in control subjects, very much in line with clinical experience, and suggesting the importance of a physical stressor in precipitating the critical autoimmune assault on the β-cell (Littorin et al. 2001).

8.3 Eating disorders

The common eating disorders associated with Type 1 diabetes are not usually 'classical' anorexia nervosa or bulimia nervosa, though a link between bulimia and Type 1 diabetes has been proposed. 'Disturbed eating behaviour' is a more appropriate term for the usual disorder seen, comprising dieting and intense exercise for weight control, binge eating, and insulin omission. Other features of classical eating disorders, such as self-induced vomiting and laxative use, are not more common in women with diabetes. However, where Type 1 diabetes and anorexia co-exist there is, not surprisingly, a very poor outlook. A standardized mortality ratio of 14.5 and a 12-yr mortality of 36% have been reported, with both acute and chronic complications contributing to death around 30 yrs of age, that is about 20 yrs after diagnosis (Walker et al. 2002). Insulin omission seems to carry an especially poor prognosis. The Joslin Clinic reported a threefold increased mortality (death occurring on average 13 yrs earlier than in women who did not restrict insulin), with higher rates of nephropathy and foot problems in an 11-yr follow-up study (Goebel-Fabbri et al. 2008). This highlights the importance of sensitive, repeated, but focused questioning on this difficult area.

It has been pointed out that there are common features shared by the classical eating disorders and desirable self-management in Type 1 diabetes—for example, attention to body weight and food portions and carbohydrate counting, and continued focusing of attention on these factors may increase the risk of eating disorders. Increased reporting of eating disorders in Type 1 diabetes coincided with the increasing acceptance of the post-DCCT model of tight glycaemic control through increased intensity of insulin treatment, increasing total insulin doses, and weight gain, with the associated risk of developing a poor body image. However, around the same time the desirability of the slim female form was emerging in popular culture, and societal and peer pressures are likely to have been important drivers behind any secular trends.

Weight loss can easily be achieved in Type 1 diabetes, first by avoiding hypoglycaemia, and second by reducing or omitting insulin. Nearly one-third of women between 13 and 60 yrs reported intentional insulin omission, up to 40% in those aged between 15 and 30. It may start at a time when parental supervision of insulin administration begins to tail off, though the triggering events may be earlier—the dramatic weight loss at onset, followed by the equally dramatic weight gain with initial insulin treatment has been proposed. Nearly 10% frequently omitted insulin, and it was surprisingly common even in older women between 45 and 60 yrs old (Polonsky et al. 1994). Practices can be extreme, and are probably under-reported, with some young women admitting taking insulin only twice a week, and even omitting it for up to 2 weeks over long periods during adolescence and early adulthood (Bryden et al. 1999). Despite this, and despite increasing concern with body weight and shape with age, females started overweight as adolescents, and mean BMI increased to 24 by their 20s. Weight gain in non-diabetic adolescents is strongly associated with recreational internet time, alcohol consumption, and lack of sleep, and these factors are also likely to contribute to weight gain in young females with diabetes. Males had similar BMI at follow-up, and gained more weight over the same period (initial BMI 20), yet eating disorders and insulin manipulation are very uncommon, so additional factors must be operating in females.

The majority of studies report A1C levels 1% to 2% higher in women with eating disorders and diabetes compared with those who do not have eating disorders, and are associated with much higher DKA rates, and markedly increased rates of microvascular complications, especially retinopathy (about 60% more prevalent in those with eating disorders than without) and neuropathy. Visceral autonomic neuropathy, especially gastroparesis, appears to be especially common in this group of young women, and can be an intractably difficult clinical situation (see Section 5.5.5.1).

Disordered eating is difficult to diagnose in Type 1 patients, and is frequently sub-threshold (though not sub-clinical). Clues include excessive concerns about weight and body shape, extreme patterns of exercise, unusual elevations of A1C, recurrent DKA, and amenorrhoea (Goebel-Fabbri et al. 2002). Prospective studies also identify greater levels of depression, decreased self-worth in relation to physical appearance, and increasing BMI in the period before onset of disturbed eating behaviour. It is very difficult in routine clinical practice to gain an idea of the proportion of insulin doses omitted; a clinical psychologist is more likely to be able to elicit this critical information, as well as other subtle features of impending trouble. Extensive questionnaires have been devised but they are too cumbersome for routine use.

Associated features include depression, associated with poor glycaemic control. It is not clear whether poor glycaemia causes depression, or vice versa—possibly the situation in Type 2 diabetes—or they may exist in a reciprocal relationship, each reinforcing the other, for example, hyperglycaemia leading to physical symptoms that then may reinforce poor self-care.

8.4 **Adolescents and young adults**

8.4.1 **Quality of life (QoL)**

QoL, indicated by broad measures of physical, psychological, and family well-being, is not surprisingly consistently reduced in adolescents. The results in narrower domains are less consistent; for example, some find problems in the formation of close personal relationships, others not. A subtle and complex matter like this, depending on a host of developmental, psychological, social, and physical characteristics, all themselves varying between individuals with (and without) diabetes is hardly likely to be consistently problematic. Overall, however, the considerable demands of self-care, often attained through significant rigour and self-discipline, frequently impact on the routine of life and impair social well-being.

It is controversial whether or not improved glycaemic control is associated with improved QoL, and if so, the direction of the causal link. In the DCCT, intensive control was associated with decreased QoL, but outside an intensive and pressured clinical trial environment, there is general agreement that good glycaemic control is associated with better QoL. For example, the international Hvidøre study also found that better control was associated with lesser perceived burden both by parents and health-care professionals. Girls, single-parent families, ethnic minorities all had worse QoL and A1C levels, and targeting these groups, perhaps with regular assessments of QoL, may be helpful (Hoey *et al.* 2001). This has been confirmed in an unselected group of adolescents, where regular assessment of QoL and detailed discussion of the results over a year improved measures of psychosocial health, behaviour, mental health, and family activities, except those in baseline poor control (A1C >9.5%); however, these limited interventions produced no overall change in glycaemic control (deWit *et al.* 2008). In recent studies, intensive diabetes treatment in children and adolescents has not been associated with impaired QoL, and when it leads to improved glycaemic control may mitigate the impact of diabetes itself on QoL. Other important findings from recent studies include the following:

- The impact of diabetes was the same in both sexes, regardless of age or duration, but was less in those with lowest A1C (7% vs 11%)
- After the age of 12 yrs, worry significantly increased in girls. Diabetes did not seem to cause as much worry to or have as much impact on patients as it did on their parents
- There was no relation between number of insulin injections a day and QoL, though higher daily insulin doses and BMI were associated with lower QoL
- Adolescents with two parents at home had a lower mean A1C compared with single-parent families (8.6% vs 9.0%), though there was no relation between family structure and QoL. Ethnic minorities had worse glycaemic control and higher worries.

8.4.2 Family functioning and dynamics

Families vary widely in their ability to cope with the stresses of diabetes. A fully engaged family team working positively on all fronts with the young diabetic person is the best environment for the management of Type 1 diabetes; not unexpectedly, these families are characterized by cohesion, good organization, and an ability to maintain a good affective environment. However, in cross-sectional studies association indicates neither causation nor direction of the causal link. At the other extreme (and with the same cautions over causation) recurrent DKA in adolescents is usually associated with significant family dysfunction, and poor adherence to insulin regimens and poor glycaemic control are associated with single parenthood and lower income and ethnic minority status. Areas of family dynamics that are likely to have a significant negative impact include:

- Conflict relating to specific diabetes problems, particularly blood glucose monitoring, which is frequently a focus of disagreement over responsibility

- Less parental involvement and greater general disagreements between the individual and their parents, which may predict poorer glycaemic outcomes
- Poor parental (especially maternal) psychological well-being
- Failure to find a balance between 'helicopter' parenting and laissez-faire
- Obsessive tendencies in parents and the young person, often resulting in creditable glycaemic control, but at the cost of low mood and anxiety. Psychological well-being and good glycaemic control are not closely correlated (Cameron et al. 2007).

Within a few years of diagnosis, up to 20% of adolescents may not be attending clinics even annually. The reasons are complex, and include lack of interest in discussing medical concerns with professionals, and an association with disrupted families and high divorce rates. These patients have worse glycaemic control and more complications than regular clinical attenders. Simplifying the logistics of making appointments and contact with the diabetes team through improved communications may materially improve this situation. In the UK, the primary care and community liaison teams could be important in encouraging defaulting Type 1 patients to resume therapeutic contact, though target-orientated management does not encourage this for the relatively small numbers of Type 1 patients.

8.4.3 **Neurocognitive functioning**

As with adults, the adolescent DCCT cohort (13- to 19-yrs old at entry) followed up in the EDIC showed no decline in cognitive function after 18-yr follow-up, despite higher rates of severe hypoglycaemia (coma or seizure) than in the adults, though psychomotor efficiency was decreased in those with higher A1C values (Musen et al. 2008). The high hypoglycaemia rates are probably due to the higher insulin doses, and the more erratic exercise and eating habits of adolescents compared with adults. The absence of significant adverse long-term neurocognitive effects contrasts with the findings in younger children, especially those diagnosed under 4 yrs, who are more likely to have decreased memory and learning capacity, associated with both severe hypo- and hyperglycaemia; those with recurrent severe hypoglycaemia had lower intellectual capacity.

While hypoglycaemia had no significant impact on neurocognitive function in DCCT/EDIC, there is some evidence for a general decline in cognitive function in Type 1 diabetes. A cross-sectional study found that long duration and early age of onset were associated with impaired performance in a wide array of neuropsychological tests—not excluding an effect of severe childhood hypoglycaemia, which was not defined in detail as it was in the DCCT/EDIC. Glycaemic control, as in many studies, was associated with electrophysiological tests of peripheral nerve function, but interestingly not with results of tests of cognitive function, which were more closely associated with non-glycaemic variables, for example obesity and hypertension (Brismar et al. 2007), a recurring theme in microvascular complications, and now hinted at in CNS involvement in long-term Type 1 diabetes.

8.4.4 Interventions

Several type of intervention have been described (counselling-based, cognitive behaviour therapy, psychoanalytical-based treatments, and family therapies), but cognitive behaviour therapy for adolescents in the family or parent group setting was the commonest form identified in a systematic review and meta-analysis (Winkley et al. 2006). The effect on A1C was modest but statistically significant (~0.5% reduction, with a mean follow-up period of 11 months), and there was a moderate effect on psychological distress. These results contrast with a much smaller, non-significant effect using similar interventions in adults, and reflect either the higher level of distress in children and their families, or a greater responsiveness to this form of intervention in the parents of young people with a chronic illness. Motivational interviewing, a relatively new and promising technique of counselling with the aim of facilitating behavioural change, has been shown to improve glycaemic control over 12 months by ~0.4% compared with a control group of teenagers. Glycaemic improvement and some measures of psychosocial functioning were maintained in the year following the end of the intervention (Channon et al. 2007), despite a lower intensity of intervention (4 vs 6 interviews).

8.5 Depression

The prevalence of major depression in young people aged 18 to 23, 10 yrs after diagnosis, was nearly 28%, nearly ten times higher in females than males, and was the most common psychiatric diagnosis in adolescence (others were conduct and generalized anxiety disorders, accounting for another 20%). Generalized anxiety disorder was characteristic of the young adults. The overall disorder rate is more than two- to threefold increased compared with the general population. Most initial depressive episodes were presumably not diagnosed, since nearly three-quarters were untreated. The recurrence rate was very high—about one-half relapsed within 6 yrs of the initial episode—though nearly one-half were treated on this occasion. Depression in these young people ends to run a more chronic course than in non-diabetic people (Kovacs et al. 1997a,b). Maternal psychopathology, especially depression, were risk factors for depression in the subjects, and parents of diabetic youngsters seem to be more aware of psychological problems in their offspring than in the general population. Specifically seeking out the diagnosis of depression in young people would seem wise, as clinical diagnosis may be masked by the physical symptoms and impaired QoL associated with poor glucose control.

There is less information on depression in adults with Type 1 diabetes, though major depression is probably more common than in non-diabetic people. Depression in adults, in contrast with adolescents and young adults, is probably more common in males, and occurs well before the onset of long-term complications. This suggestion does not preclude the possibility of biological—as opposed to psychosocial—mediators between Type 1 diabetes and depression (more strongly hinted at in Type 2 diabetes). Some of the features of poorly controlled diabetes, for example, fatigue, daytime somnolence, weight loss, and nocturnal wakening, may also be features of depression, but affective symptoms (low mood, anhedonism, anxiety, shame, fear) are more likely to be depressive in origin (Jacobson 2004). Self-care may be compromised in some patients with depression, as in patients with tissue complications, for example, retinopathy or cataracts impairing visual function, or erectile dysfunction; successful treatment may allow improved self-care to re-emerge.

8.6 **Tissue complications**

Complications are associated with a two- to threefold increased rate of depressive disorders. More intriguing, in a large mixed group of Type 1 and Type 2 patients with a first foot ulcer, both major and minor depressive disorders—prevalence 25% and 8%, respectively—tripled the risk of death over 18 months. The causal links are not clear: lack of adherence to the medical regimen, behavioural difficulties, problems with self-care, and intervening events, such as amputation, do not fully explain the increased risk, and several organic mediators, for example autonomic neuropathy, cytokine responses, and abnormalities of the ACTH–cortisol axis may play an as yet undetermined role. However, regardless of the causation, these findings reinforce the important role of active diagnosis and management of depression in patients with complications (Ismail et al. 2007). The high prevalence of erectile dysfunction, occurring at a relatively early age in Type 1 diabetes, and sometimes resistant to standard PDE5 inhibitor treatment, is a common cause of severe depression.

References

Brismar T, Maurex L, Cooray G et al. (2007). Predictors of cognitive impairment in type 1 diabetes. *Psychoneuroendocrinology*, **32**: 1041–51. [PMID: 17884300]

Bryden KS, Neil A, Mayou RA, Peveler RC, Fairburn CG, Dunger DB (1999). Eating habits, body weight, and insulin misuse. A longitudinal study of teenagers and young adults with type 1 diabetes. *Diabetes Care*, **22**: 1956–60. [PMID: 10587825]

Cameron FJ, Northam EA, Ambler GR, Daneman D (2007). Routine psychological screening in youth with type 1 diabetes and their parents: a notion whose time has come? *Diabetes Care*, **30**: 2716–24. [PMID: 17644619]

Channon SJ, Huws-Thomas MV, Rollnick S et al. (2007). A multicenter randomized controlled trial of motivational interviewing in teenagers with diabetes. *Diabetes Care*, **30**: 1390–5. [PMID: 17351283]

Goebel-Fabbri AE, Fikkan J, Connell A, Vangsness L, Anderson BJ (2002). Identification and treatment of eating disorders in women with type 1 diabetes mellitus. *Treat Endocrinol*, **1**: 155–62. [PMID: 15799208]

Goebel-Fabbri AE, Fikkan J, Franko DL, Pearson K, Anderson BJ, Weinger K (2008). Insulin restriction and associated morbidity and mortality in women with type 1 diabetes. *Diabetes Care*, **31**: 415–9. [PMID: 18070998]

Hoey H, Aanstoot HJ, Chiarelli F et al. (2001). Good metabolic control is associated with better quality of life in 2101 adolescents with type 1 diabetes. *Diabetes Care*, **24**: 1923–8. [PMID: 11679458]

Ismail K, Winkley K, Stahil D, Chalder T, Edmonds M (2007). A cohort study of people with diabetes and their first foot ulcer: the role of depression on mortality. *Diabetes Care*, **30**: 1473–9. [PMID: 17363754]

Jacobson AM (2004). Psychological problems and management of patients with diabetes mellitus. Chapter 91 in: *International Textbook of Diabetes Mellitus*, 3rd edn. DeFronzo R, Ferrannini E, Keen H, Zimmet P (eds). John Wiley & Sons. ISBN: 978-0-47-148655-8

Kovacs M, Goldston D, Obrosky DS, Bonar LK (1997a). Psychiatric disorders in youths with IDDM: rates and risk factors. *Diabetes Care*, **20**: 36–44. [PMID: 9028691]

Kovacs M, Obrosky DS, Goldston D, Drash A (1997b). Major depressive disorder in youths with IDDM. A controlled prospective study of course and outcome. *Diabetes Care*, **20**: 45–51. [PMID: 9028692]

Littorin B, Sundkvist G, Nyström L et al.; Diabetes Incidence Study in Sweden (DISS) (2001). Family characteristics and life events before the onset of autoimmune type 1 diabetes in young adults: a nationwide study. *Diabetes Care*, **24**: 1033–7. [PMID: 11375366]

Musen G, Jacobson AM, Ryan CM et al.; The DCCT/EDIC Research Group (2008). The impact of diabetes and its treatment on cognitive function among adolescents who participated in the DCCT. *Diabetes Care*, **31**: 1933–8. [PMID: 18606979]

Polonsky WH, Anderson BJ, Lohrer PA, Aponte JE, Jacobson AM, Cole CF (1994). Insulin omission in women with IDDM. *Diabetes Care*, **17**: 1178–85. [PMID: 7821139]

Walker JD, Young RJ, Little J, Steel JM (2002). Mortality in concurrent type 1 diabetes and anorexia nervosa. *Diabetes Care*, **25**: 1664–5. [PMID: 12196451]

Winkley K, Ismail K, Landau S, Eisler I (2006). Psychological interventions to improve glycaemic control in patients with type 1 diabetes: systematic review and meta-analysis of randomised controlled trials. *BMJ*, **333**: 65. [PMID: 16803942]

deWit M, Delemaare-van de Waal HA, Bokma JA *et al.* (2008). Monitoring and discussing health-related quality of life in adolescents with type 1 diabetes improve psychosocial well-being: a randomized controlled trial. *Diabetes Care*, **31**: 1521–6. [PMID: 18509204]

Further reading

Anderson BJ, Rubin RR (eds) (2002). *Practical Psychology for Diabetes Clinicians*, 2nd revised edn. American Diabetes Association. ISBN: 978–1–58–040140-1

Chapter 9

Practical matters

9.1 Blood glucose monitoring

Self-monitoring of blood glucose (SMBG) first became practical in the late 1970s when blood glucose testing technology (strips and meters, initially colorimetric) was first developed. Capillary glucose measurements can now be made in a few seconds using tiny samples, and the achievement of near-normoglycaemia with intensive insulin therapy in a substantial proportion of Type 1 patients is in large part a result of SMBG.

In contrast with Type 2 diabetes, there is no controversy about the benefits of SMBG in Type 1 diabetes or the establishment of individual targets for blood glucose levels. In the intensively treated group of the Diabetes Control and Complications Trial (DCCT), SMBG was recommended ≥4 times daily, with a night-time measurement at least weekly, and three or more measurements daily were made on ~90% of days throughout the study (see Section 5.2.2). Most importantly, adjustments to insulin doses were made in the vast majority of intensive patients on the basis of SMBG. Because of the multiple interventions in the intensive DCCT group, it is not possible to determine the absolute benefit of SMBG, and no RCTs will be performed in Type 1 diabetes, but one study found that glycaemic control deteriorated when fewer than four daily measurements were made, and increased frequency of SMBG and insulin injections are associated with, though not necessarily causally related to, lower A1C.

Data accumulated in glucose meters, often in very large quantities, must be presented in a meaningful way that does not overload the acquirer or the diabetes team. The traditional written logbook format is still probably the best way to recognize patterns of glucose excursions, and especially their variability, in relation to meals, though download software and apps for mobile devices have made the process less laborious. Motivating patients to move from zero to any systematic SMBG is difficult but important; even the single random capillary glucose measurement traditionally taken at a diabetes clinic attendance can be used as an educational tool in the person not performing SMBG—and if the measurement is post-lunch, it correlates reasonably well with A1C levels.

9.1.1 Continuous glucose monitoring (CGM)

This is another area where 'pure' technology has benefited people with Type 1 diabetes. It is important to distinguish between the diagnostic and therapeutic roles of CGM. Earlier devices were not real time, were intended only for occasional use, and therefore were only diagnostic. A new generation of inexpensive wireless monitoring systems with real-time display of (interstitial) glucose measurements is currently being introduced, and it is possible that they may replace SMBG as a therapeutic tool (Figure 9.1). However, even the most recent of these devices has a delay of ~15 min, of which about one-half represents the expected physiological delay between changes in blood and interstitial glucose levels, and the remainder by instrumental processing delays (Wei et al. 2010). Evidence is now accumulating on the benefits of near-permanent CGM. In a representative group of patients, poorly controlled on MDI (A1C 9.2–9.4%) and moving to CSII, using the sensor >70% of the time further improved A1C over 6 months by ~0.4% (though most of the overall improvement (1.2%) was due to the change from MDI to CSII). It remains to be seen whether long-term adherence to this technology is clinically practical, maintains the short-term improvements, and reduces the risk of severe hypoglycaemia and DKA (Raccah et al. 2009). The Juvenile Diabetes Research Foundation has done a thorough 6 month randomised trial of CGM in patients of all ages. These very promptly-conducted studies now give sound initial guidance for the use of this important new technique:

- Glycaemia improved by ~0.5% in adults 25 yrs or older so long as CGM was used for 6 days a week or more. Younger people between 8 and 25 yrs did not seem to gain glycaemic benefit
- Severe hypoglycaemic episodes fell in patients of all ages if A1C was 7.0% or more (JDRF CGM Study group 2008 and 2010a). Diagnostic CGM for occasional use should be widely available (see Section 4.2). It has confirmed that in real life:
- Stable glucose levels are rarely attained (though this situation can now be approximated with CSII)
- Nocturnal hypoglycaemia (glucose <3.3 mmol/L) is equally common with CSII and MDI, and episodes lasting at least 20 mins

occur about every 14 nights; nearly one-quarter of all episodes last 2 hrs or more. This is another caution against the automatic assumption that 'modern' insulin technology automatically reduces the most serious complication of Type 1 diabetes (JDRF CGM Study Group 2010b).

- Blood glucose can rise very rapidly to high values after meals, even with rapid-acting analogues, and allowing for the delay in interstitial, compared with blood, glucose measurements
- Patterns of glycaemia are much easier to detect than with even frequent SMBG; where there are rapid changes in glucose levels, small differences in the timing of insulin injections and SMBG can give the impression of greater glucose variability than there actually is.

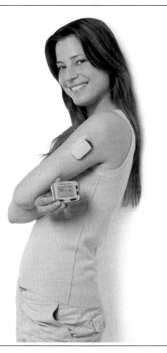

Figure 9.1 Freestyle Navigator CGM system. The sensor is attached to the upper arm or abdomen, and transmits interstitial glucose levels to the receiver every minute. Data are transmitted wirelessly to the receiver, which stores and displays glucose data. Trends in glucose levels can be displayed graphically, arrows indicate current trends, and alarms can be set for high or low glucose values. Audio warnings can be set to anticipate pre-selected glucose levels and to warn of impending hypoglycaemia. The sensor life is 5 days. Photograph courtesy of Abbott.

9.2 **Exercise**

Exercise increases the risk of hypoglycaemia, but is critically important for general health and for maintaining cardiovascular fitness. It is also an important part of the educational and social progress of young people, and managing its complexities is a priority so that Type 1 patients can safely undertake regular and ad lib exercise. As in the general population, every attempt should be made to achieve the target of 30 min moderate-intensity exercise at least five times a week.

There is relatively little evidence on the physiology and even less on the management of glycaemia during and after exercise in Type 1 diabetes. However, it is helpful to distinguish between three varieties of exercise, which seem to generate different glucoregulatory responses:

- *Moderate-intensity exercise* (continuous aerobic activity, e.g. running/jogging, cycling, swimming—55% to 70% maximum heart rate). This generally causes a fall in blood glucose, due to high unchanging circulating insulin suppressing hepatic glucose production. In addition, glucagon-stimulated hepatic gluconeogenesis, an important determinant of increased glucose levels in non-diabetic individuals in this type of activity, is attenuated in Type 1 diabetes. Hypoglycaemia has been reported to occur up to 17 to 30 h after moderate exercise, through continuing muscle and liver requirements to replenish glycogen via non-oxidative glucose disposal. Of more immediate concern, especially in adolescents, increased glucose disposal occurs 7 to 11 h after exercise, and this may be due to an intriguing phenomenon of impaired counter-regulatory responses caused by sleep itself (it occurs in young non-diabetic people as well) (Tamborlane 2007). Exercising in the late evening therefore carries a greatly increased risk of nocturnal hypoglycaemia. General advice is to reduce the prior fast-acting insulin dose by 25%, and supplementing with 15 to 30 g rapidly acting carbohydrate (CHO) every 30 min for exercise lasting an hour or less; for prolonged exercise, for example long-distance running, up to 70% to 80% reduction in insulin dose is recommended. In pump-treated patients, simply discontinuing the basal infusion just before exercise at least halves the risk of hypoglycaemia. The hypoglycaemia associated with moderate-intensity exercise is attenuated by just one 10-s burst of maximum sprinting before exercise, and, though counterintuitive, suggest exercising in the fasting state first thing in the morning, when circulating insulin levels are likely to be low, rather than the more risky though more conventional late afternoon–early evening.

- *High-intensity exercise* (sports involving sprints or repeated short bursts of intense activity >75% maximum heart rate). This is usually considered to be 'anaerobic' exercise, almost exclusively through metabolism of glucose and glycogen (not fatty acids, metabolism of which is aerobic). Importantly, blood glucose levels rise during and even after this form of exercise, largely because of increased catecholamine production. Appropriate management would be to increase insulin doses slightly where this is a consistent feature (Marliss and Vranic 2002).

Intermittent high-intensity exercise. A hybrid that resembles much real-life exercise—short bursts of high-intensity exercise, often lasting only a few seconds, alternating either with rest or moderate-intensity exercise (e.g. many team and field sports, and spontaneous play in children). In general, glucose levels drop during this kind of activity, but to a lesser extent than in moderate-intensity exercise, again probably mediated through high catecholamine levels. The reductions in insulin doses and CHO supplementation recommended for moderate-intensity exercise might not be appropriate here (Guelfi *et al.* 2007).

These studies and recommendations are based on younger Type 1 patients without complications and, importantly, without hypoglycaemia unawareness or hypoglycaemia-induced autonomic failure. Documenting blood glucose responses to exercise in individual patients will help individualize management—but recognising that hypoglycaemia is not the only glucose response to activity is important. Members of diabetes teams usually strenuously avoid discussing sexual activity and its effects on glucose levels, but anxiety to avoid hypoglycaemia under these circumstances may encourage deliberate nocturnal hyperglycaemia, especially in young people. Substantial dose reductions both of evening meal short-acting and where appropriate bedtime long-acting insulin, according to circumstances, would be obvious strategies—reports of unexpected nocturnal hypoglycaemia should prompt sensitive questioning.

Unravelling the complex, probably reciprocal, relationship between exercise and long-term complications requires a long-term prospective study. In a cross-sectional study in Type 1 patients, nephropathy, advanced retinopathy, and cardiovascular disease were, not surprisingly, associated with physical inactivity, but even patients with microalbuminuria, presumably in the absence of significant exercise-limiting factors, also reported lower levels of leisure-time activity—hinting that lower activity may be causally related to microalbuminuria (Wadén *et al.* 2008).

9.3 Infections

There is a debate whether or not well-controlled Type 1 diabetes is associated with an increased risk of bacterial infections. Countless experimental studies have demonstrated defects in host defences in both Type 1 and Type 2 diabetes, but there is no evidence that there are innate immune abnormalities in Type 1 diabetes that predispose to infection—the metabolic abnormalities and hyperglycaemia appear to account fully for the predisposition. A very large study in Dutch primary care confirms a 1.5- to 2-fold increased risk of several common infections in Type 1 patients, for example:

- Lower respiratory infections
- Urinary tract infections
- Bacterial skin and mucous membrane infections
- Fungal skin and mucous membrane infections (Muller *et al.* 2005).

There is an overall fourfold increased risk of pneumonia, but the risk is increased even in young people with A1C levels <7%. Influenza and pneumococcal immunizations are therefore important in all Type 1 patients, and appear to be as effective as in non-diabetic people. However, adequate protective antibody responses to hepatitis B vaccines are lower in Type 1 diabetes.

Urinary tract infections are probably more common in women with Type 1 diabetes than non-diabetic women. Risk increases with duration and A1C. Longer antibiotic treatment protocols should be used because of the tendency to involve the upper urinary tract, and patients with systemic symptoms should be admitted for intravenous antibiotics and monitoring of glycaemia.

The very rare, though life-threatening, infections considered 'specific' to diabetes, including rhinocerebral mucormycosis and 'malignant' otitis externa, should always be remembered, but in clinical practice it is the common organisms, especially *Staphylococcus aureus* (sensitive or methicillin-resistant *S. aureus* [MRSA]) and streptococci occurring in unusual sites that frequently elude detection. Remote osteomyelitis, septic arthritis, and spinal and intra-abdominal infections are recurring traps, especially in patients with advanced complications, where pain may not be fully percieved as a result of neuropathy.

9.4 **Alcohol**

The general recommendations for alcohol intake apply to people with Type 1 diabetes, but safe management of alcohol requires careful education, especially in relation to hypoglycaemia. Hypoglycaemia and alcohol are linked in several ways (Richardson *et al.* 2005):

- Hypoglycaemia awareness may be impaired by alcohol
- Alcohol may impair counter-regulatory responses to hypoglycaemia, and also further impair cognition already reduced by hypoglycaemia
- Hypoglycaemia associated with alcohol is a common reason for hospital attendances in insulin-treated people (up to 20% in an early study from the 1980s).

he conventional view on the relationship between alcohol and ucose levels is that moderate alcohol taken alone has little effect cutely, but increases the risk of hypoglycaemia the next day. The esults of CGM studies are not consistent. Alcohol taken with a candard meal overall reduced interstitial glucose levels by 1.2 imol/L, and was associated with double the frequency of hypogly-aemia during the following 24 h. A more real-life study of moder-tely heavy social alcohol consumption in Australian adolescents ver a 12-h period during a weekend night (social here means an verage of nine drinks in males, six in females) was associated with icreased glucose variability, but not hypoglycaemia (Ismail et al. 006). These results underline the variable responses to alcohol eported by individual patients, but it would be wise to err on the de of caution in warning about the risks of late hypoglycaemia—ven when taken with adequate CHO.

The combination of moderate hypoglycaemia (2.3 mmol/L) and ufficient alcohol to result in blood alcohol levels below the UK riving limit caused especially marked cognitive impairment, and ype 1 patients should be strongly advised to avoid all alcohol if riving (Cheyne et al. 2004). More encouragingly, in cross-sectional ata from the EURODIAB complications study, moderate alcohol onsumption (30 to 70 g/week, ~2 to 5 drinks, especially wine) was ssociated with a significantly lower risk of microvascular complica-ons (proliferative retinopathy, neuropathy, and macroalbuminuria). lowever in this study, acute complications (DKA and severe hypog-rcaemia) were not associated with alcohol consumption (Beulens et . 2008), though alcohol emerges as a frequent precipitant of DKA in iost studies (see Section 2.6.1).

9.5 **Driving**

i early analyses, insulin-treated patients were found to be at increased sk of moving vehicle violations. A more recent international survey, onducted after publication of DCCT and UKPDS, found that in both ie USA and Europe, a wider range of driving mishaps (crashes, viola-ons, stupor, requiring assistance, and symptomatic hypoglycaemia) ccurred in Type 1 diabetes (mean age 42 yrs, mean duration 18 to 22 rs) than in Type 2 or spouse controls (but overall risk was still only pout half that associated with other long-term conditions that do not urrently attract medical restrictions, e.g. attention-deficit hyperactivity sorder, sleep apnoea, alcohol abuse). Severe hypoglycaemia while riving was less common in Europe than USA, possibly because of the tringency of licence renewal procedures in Europe—typically every yrs, and more frequently if problems have been identified (Box 9.1). he same study found, alarmingly, that only one-half of Type 1 patients reported discussing hypoglycaemia and driving with their physicians, though about one-third of UK drivers admitted that they had experienced hypoglycaemia. Long-term complications, especially neuropathy and retinopathy, are not considered to be significant risk factors, but insulin pump treatment is significantly associated with hypoglycaemia while driving (Cox et al. 2009). It is interesting to speculate on the reasons for this finding, which needs further exploration as pump treatment becomes much more widespread. Patients with visual impairment from any cause tend to give up driving (and in many countries patients with diabetes require visual acuity testing; Cox et al. 2003).

Safe driving requires close attention, rapid reactions, and high levels of motor coordination, and therefore is continuously under scrutiny as an activity that might be impaired by hypoglycaemia. Even so, reported accident rates may be an insensitive measure of more frequent day-to-day impairment of driving technique, transient episodes of minor impairment of attention and consciousness, and consequent minor accidents that are not formally reported. In support of this, but extending the range of problems into a more serious category, a survey from the USA found that annually 40% of Type 1 patients reported disruptive hypoglycaemia where the subjects could still treat themselves, but no longer drive safely. Importantly, 18% disclosed an episode of automatic driving resulting in disorientation or arriving at their destination with no recollection of driving there (Cox et al. 2009).

Perception of risk must also be taken into account: young non-diabetic males, in particular, tend to underestimate their risk of having an accident, while overestimating their skill. Few studies have assessed the perception of risk and ability to drive safely in Type 1 patients—critical insights that may be responsible for the generally safe record of Type 1 diabetic patients who drive. However, experimental clamp studies with extensive neuropsychological testing found:

- As blood glucose levels fell, fewer subjects reported that they felt safe about driving, but
- 20% to 40% of patients judged they were safe to drive with blood glucose levels ≤2.8 mmol/L
- Factors associated with increasing awareness of risk included: female gender, young age, accurate self-estimation of blood glucose levels, and cognitive impairment.

The age relationship contrasts with the finding in non-diabetic subjects and may be related to several factors, for example older Type 1 patients may be more experienced drivers and more likely to be confident while driving when hypoglycaemic; medical teams are more likely to reinforce education about driving safety with younger diabetic people; and hypoglycaemia unawareness increases with diabetes duration (Boxes 9.1 and 9.2) (Weinger et al. 1999).

150

In practice, nearly all UK drivers inform the licensing authority and insurers about insulin treatment. Most were aware that blood glucose levels of 4.0 mmol/L or more were necessary for safe driving, and kept CHO in their vehicle (Graveling *et al.* 2004). However, in the same study, nearly 40% did not keep a glucose meter in their vehicle, 60% never tested blood glucose before driving, and most relied on symptoms of hypoglycaemia during driving rather than blood glucose measurements. Factual information is being given (though physicians do not seem to be doing it very effectively), but delivering consistent and detailed information that is retained and implemented in real life is less successful (Box 9.2).

Box 9.1 Practical aspects of driving licensing in UK (after Frier 2007)

- Mandatory disclosure of insulin requirement to licensing authority (DVLA) and insurers
- Relicensing required at least every 3 yrs; general practitioner, specialist reports required
- Vans and lorries (3.5–7.5 tonnes; C1 licence) can be driven for employment purposes; requirements are more stringent, and annual clinical reviews needed
- In Europe, except the UK, D1 licences can be granted to drive mini-buses carrying up to 16 passengers for employment purposes; in the UK, voluntary driving of mini-buses is permitted
- Large goods vehicles (LGV) and passenger-carrying vehicles (PCV)—licences not permitted for insulin-treated drivers
- Licensed cabs—at the discretion of individual licensing authorities

---

Box 9.2 Practical advice for drivers on prevention and management of hypoglycaemia

- Check blood glucose levels before even short journeys
- Measure regularly, e.g. two-hourly during longer journeys
- Take frequent snacks and rest stops; do not drink alcohol
- Have ready access to fast-acting CHO (sweets, glucose) in the vehicle at all times; anticipate traffic delays (GPS might be helpful) and unexpected activity, e.g. changing a wheel, which may require longer-acting CHO
- If symptomatically hypoglycaemic:
  - Pull over in a safe place, remove keys from ignition
  - Move to passenger seat to avoid the possibility of being charged with driving under the influence of a drug, i.e. insulin
  - Take appropriate glucose
  - Do not drive again for 45 min (time required for full recovery of cognitive function after restoration of normal blood glucose level)

151

9.6 **Diet and carbohydrate counting**

The primary goals of nutrition therapy in Type 1 diabetes include:

- Balancing specific dietary recommendations with the restrictions of insulin therapy
- Minimizing hypoglycaemia, while
  - ensuring optimum growth and development in young people
  - reducing the adverse metabolic and cardiovascular effects of acquired insulin resistance.

However, there is limited randomized controlled trial (RCT) evidence for any specific dietary approaches to achieve these goals.

The CHO content of food is the major determinant of bolus insulin doses, and CHO counting based on the CHO exchange system has been used for decades, usually inflexibly and with fixed insulin regimens (though many older people with long-standing uncomplicated Type 1 diabetes attribute their good health to the rigid and monotonous dietary regimens instilled in them by their mothers). However, with basal-bolus insulin regimens in the 1980s, greater dietary flexibility became possible, with potential for improved glycaemic control at the same time. While Type 1 patients have undoubtedly greater dietary flexibility, there is scant evidence for overall improved glycaemic control in larger groups of people with Type 1 diabetes (see Sections 7.4.1 and 7.4.2), though achieving flexibility without significant deterioration in glycaemia should be considered a significant achievement. For example, a study of simple CHO counting based on 10 g portion size, not taking into account refinements such as glycaemic index, fibre, lipid, and calorie content of meals, maintained good glycaemic control without hypoglycaemia on both high- and low-CHO diets, provided individuals can accurately estimate CHO content (Rabasa-Lhoret *et al.* 1999). The impact of non-CHO aspects of diet has not been explored in detail, though higher fatty acid and lower fibre consumption was associated with retinopathy progression in the DCCT.

9.6.1 **Dietary composition—DCCT and beyond**

In the intensively treated DCCT CHO counting was associated with an additional fall of 0.5% A1C. Although the intensive group had frequent and detailed dietary input (at least monthly dietetic visits for the first 6 months), dietary composition goals, which were also established in the conventional group, were subverted to the primacy of good glycaemic control in this proof-of-concept study, and the importance of dietary consistency, especially with CHOs, and meal regularity (15 to 45 min after prandial insulin) was emphasized. Accordingly, diet composition in the two groups turned out to be nearly identical (median calories 2330; 45% calories from CHO, 18% from protein, 38% from fat [13% saturated], cholesterol 400 mg/day, dietary fibre 26 g/day; DCCT Research Group 2005). Current recommendations are for rather lower amounts of saturated fat (<7% vs 13%) and cholesterol (<200 mg/day vs 400 mg/day), and higher fibre (~50 g/day vs 26 g/day; American Diabetes Association 2008).

Interest in glycaemic index is increasing in Type 1 diabetes, especially in relation to postprandial glucose regulation, which remains a problem for many people using multiple dose insulin (MDI), in spite of intensive SMBG, Dose Adjustment For Normal Eating (DAFNE)-style interventions, and fast-acting insulin analogues, and which may be especially evident on CGM. (Insulin pumps have specific programmed bolus patterns, e.g. dual wave, to help manage this particular problem; see Section 4.5.2.) Lower glycaemic index meals reduce postprandial glucose peaks in children (and fast-acting analogues should certainly be given before, and not after such meals).

9.6.2 Intensive dietary education programmes

Implementing sophisticated CHO counting strategies in routine clinical practice outside the trial setting, and evaluating their effects on glycaemic outcome and measurements of well-being is relatively recent. An intensive inpatient training programme widespread in Germany was adapted in the UK as a 5-day course, DAFNE (DAFNE Study Group 2002), whose main aim is to encourage confidence to self-adjust prandial insulin doses to desired foods, rather than adapt diet components to fixed insulin doses, by introducing (or reintroducing) simple CHO counting/estimating and the use of insulin:CHO ratios. A1C fell by 1.0% 6 months, and 0.5% 12 months after the course, but the most convincing outcomes were in general well-being, treatment satisfaction, and, at 1 yr, quality of life. The programme is now available in the UK, and widespread implementation is likely to be cost-effective. Variants have been reported in other countries, with broadly similar outcomes; a striking general finding is that beneficial effects persist up to at least a year, despite the single intervention without systematic follow-up. Consistent glycaemic benefit has been shown in countrywide evaluations: for example, a year after the course, mean A1C was reduced by 0.7%, together with a significant reduction in severe hypoglycaemia, in a long-term assessment of the original 5-day inpatient programme in nearly 100 German centres. These impressive results are probably related as much to rigorous monitoring of the nationwide programme and the associated quality-control procedures as to the programme content itself (Sämann et al. 2005).

9.7 The elderly Type 1 patient

This is an important group of people, though the literature is thin. Life expectancy of patients with Type 1 diabetes has improved. Celebrating 50 yrs of insulin-treated diabetes, often without severe complications, is now unremarkable, a 60-yr medal (named after RD Lawrence) has been instituted by the national diabetes association, Diabetes UK, and receiving the 70-yr Macleod medal will soon be a common event (see Section 5.6). The characteristics of the 50-yr survivors hints at some of their difficulties, which should not be underestimated just because they have had many preceding years of apparently trouble-free diabetes:

- They often require low or very low doses of insulin, and some may require pen devices delivering in ½ unit steps
- Educating on dosage self-adjustment is difficult in a group of people diagnosed in an era of autocratic and prescriptive diabetes management. As hypoglycaemia unawareness and the incidence of severe hypoglycaemia increases, increased, not decreased, flexibility is required
- Visual disability is common, frequently not considered, and may be very long-standing, for example in people who had laser treatment many years ago. Additional causes of gradually deteriorating vision, related to diabetes or otherwise (e.g. glaucoma, cataract, and age-related macular degeneration, of which the last is by far the commonest reason for both blind and partial sight registration in the UK) should be carefully assessed. Give careful and detailed consideration to appropriate equipment e.g. insulin pens with digital dosage displays, one of which recalls previous doses and the time they were given (HumaPen Memoir®, Lilly); speaking blood glucose meters; and meters with large displays and high contrast.
- Advanced neuropathy affecting the hands, diabetic cheiroarthropathy, and other non-diabetic rheumatological problems may prevent patients giving their own insulin injections, many of which can be overcome with the wide variety of devices currently available
- Some patients have severe glycaemic instability with very marked and rapid fluctuations of blood glucose levels (see below). These are often exacerbated by poor or erratic appetite; some elderly people continue an inappropriate and rigidly controlled diet, even when there is recurrent hypoglycaemia.

9.7.1 **Hypoglycaemia**

The clinical impression is that even low insulin doses in elderly patients with longstanding diabetes have a long effective duration of action. Managing long-acting insulin is particularly difficult; long-acting analogues appear to have similarly unpredictable effects as NPH, and are not always preferable to older insulins or even animal insulin preparations, still used and preferred by some older people. Even rapid-acting analogues seem to have a prolonged action with a tendency to produce late hypoglycaemia. The causative injection, many hours from the time of administration, may not be apparent without careful analysis.

Hypoglycaemia is an ever-present and major risk, but is not always perceived as a greater risk than moderate hyperglycaemia. Healthcare professionals who hold these views must be educated by the diabetes team that many elderly people are at greater risk of severe harm or death from hypoglycaemia than progression of microvascular complications, which many of these patients have avoided.

Hypoglycaemia risk increases with duration, is associated with increasing prevalence of hypoglycaemia unawareness, and is exacerbated by progressing small- and large-vessel cerebrovascular disease.

9.7.2 **Other factors**

- *Falls, fractures, and other injuries.* Elderly Type 1 patients are often not overweight, and may be at greater risk of fractures if they fall while hypoglycaemic. Severe hypoglycaemia-associated injuries are common and can be life-threatening (Box 9.3, Figure 9.2). Type 1 diabetes is associated with osteoporosis, and Vitamin D insufficiency or deficiency is extremely common in the UK. Both are likely to be important factors increasing the risk of falls and fractures. Screen with bone density scans and Vitamin D levels—and treat.

- *Increasing risk of autonomic neuropathy* and postural hypotension, exacerbated by medication (antihypertensives, especially diuretics and vasodilators, but not forgetting angiotensin receptor blockers, and tricyclic antidepressants)

- *Living environment.* Many have lost their life partners who may have administered insulin, cooked, and monitored their blood glucose levels for many years, often with great skill and a level of intuition that is difficult to transfer to institutional carers

- *Institutional homes.* It must be made clear to carers that management of these relatively uncommon patients is quite different from that of the much more numerous insulin-treated Type 2 patients. The absolute insulin-dependency, though often with apparently very low insulin requirements, is an important educational point; in addition, the need for more frequent blood glucose testing and the risks of hypoglycaemia and DKA must be reinforced

- *Associated conditions.* Many people with long duration Type 1 diabetes have additional autoimmune diseases—the impression is that these, especially Addison's disease (with the added complexity of rapid onsets and offsets of insulin resistance and sensitivity with frequent glucocorticoid dosing, interacting with MDI), are especially unstable.

Box 9.3 Case history—severe unpredictable hypoglycaemia ending independent home life in an elderly patient with 'brittle diabetes'

Female aged 80, Type 1 diabetes 36 yrs. She had unstable diabetes, despite usual A1C measurements ~7.5%. While living alone at home with no support, she had a severe nocturnal hypoglycaemic reaction, falling against a hot radiator. She was unconscious for several hours and suffered extensive third degree burns of the left thigh, requiring plastic procedures, and a hospital stay of 12 weeks. After multiple changes of insulin regimen while in hospital, and a reduction in the frequency of hypoglycaemia, she was discharged with home support, reliably self-administering twice-daily long-acting analogue insulin, but was readmitted the following week after another hypoglycaemic reaction. She had been unconscious for several hours before being found by her sister. In hospital there was continuing instability of blood glucose levels on the twice-daily long-acting analogue, with severe unpredictable hypoglycaemia and unawareness. Twice-daily fixed mixture insulin reduced the frequency of hypoglycaemia, but blood glucose levels were consistently in double figures. She moved from hospital to sheltered accommodation (Figure 9.2).

Figure 9.2 Photo of above patient (Box 9.3)—extensive healed burns on left thigh and leg, with skin graft donor site on right thigh

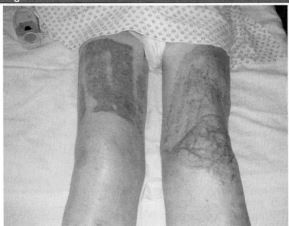

9.7.3 **Brittle diabetes in older patients**

An uncommon but very difficult situation. Unlike brittle diabetes in young women, there are no clear-cut clinical characteristics. Duration is inevitably long, with a female preponderance—this is probably a survivor effect, though both genders are equally represented in surveys of long-duration Type 1 patients (see Section 5.6). Most patients have a combination of hypoglycaemia and DKA. There are usually multiple causes, though the factors that at first sight might be thought responsible, for example hypoglycaemia unawareness, memory or behavioural problems, or deliberate manipulation appear to be relatively uncommon. Other chronic diseases and living alone may be associated factors. Hospital admissions are frequent and long (Benbow *et al.* 2001). There may be simple explanations, for example a spouse who normally gives insulin to their partner may have developed a condition that impairs their ability to continue injecting—but in practice the condition seems to be one of increasing diabetes instability that responds poorly to changing insulin types and regimens (Box 9.3).

9.8 **A1C and estimated average glucose (eAG) values**

9.8.1 **History**

Introduced into clinical practice in the early 1980s, the A1C measurement has become the standard indicator of glycaemic control. Non-enzymatic glycation of haemoglobin was discovered almost accidentally in the early 1960s, but it took a futher 15 yrs for its clinical utility in diabetes to become established (Kahn and Fonseca 2008). The DCCT established a centralized and standardized assay (using ion-exchange high-performance liquid chromatography) that has become the reference for nearly all commercial assays.

9.8.2 **More recent developments**

Two issues, one methodological, the other practical, have emerged in recent years:

• *Methodological.* Clinical biochemists prefer absolute measurements to the current percentage measure used for A1C. A highly sophisticated absolute measurement of A1C—millimoles of A1C per mole of total haemoglobin—is now possible using mass spectrometry (though routine clinical laboratory measurements will still have to be standardized rather than measured directly because of its complexity and expense; the values will be substantially lower than those using current methods). The interim solution, to be implemented fully from mid-2011, has been to convert DCCT-aligned percentage measurements to the new IFCC (International Federation of Clinical

157

Chemistry) values. Eventually the reference range will be moved down when the new standard is introduced. While technically sound, the change from the now intuitively-understood DCCT measurements—and equally importantly, shifts in the measurement, which are especially relevant to Type 1 patients—poses a major educational challenge to patients and professionals alike.

• *Practical.* Relating the percentage DCCT-aligned A1C to 'real' measurements as made by patients (mmol/L, mg/dL). SMBG data in the DCCT allowed the first practically useful correlation between eAG and A1C. This relationship has now been refined in an extensive study of non-diabetic subjects and people with both Type 1 and Type 2 diabetes, yielding thousands of glucose measurements obtained by CGMS and fingerprick. There is a close statistical correlation between eAG and A1C ($R^2 = 0.84$; Nathan *et al.* 2008), and it is recommended that a simple regression equation (eAG (mmol/L) = $1.59 \times$ A1C-2.59) should be widely used to present this additional measurement in laboratory reports. The residual variance (~16% to 19%) may be accounted for by methodological variation, but there is some concern that the relationship may be less reliable in children (variation of up to 3 mmol/L for a given A1C) and in ethnic minorities. Patients' and professionals' understanding of blood glucose variability would be enhanced if the confidence interval for the point estimate of eAG were simultaneously quoted.

9.8.3 Glycaemic variability

Several studies, including an independent analysis of the publicly available DCCT data, propose that the greater glucose variability associated with 'conventional' treatment might carry a higher risk of complications, including macrovascular complications, independent of A1C levels. A complex reanalysis of the DCCT data comparing patients with similar A1C levels in the conventional and intensive groups confirms that retinopathy risks with time are identical in the two groups, regardless of treatment allocation (Lachin *et al.* 2008). Statistically 96% of the treatment group effect is explained by differences in mean A1C; only a trivial component can be explained by the treatment group itself. For practical purposes, attained A1C regardless of the means by which it is achieved determines microvascular risk. There is still a suggestion, however, that macrovascular events in the DCCT cohort may be better predicted by glycaemic variability than A1C, and that increased variability of A1C itself, especially in the conventionally treated group, may be related to the risk of retinopathy (Kilpatrick *et al.* 2008). While academically interesting, it is of no practical relevance to the individual Type 1 patient.

References

Benbow SJ, Walsh A, Gill GV (2001). Brittle diabetes in the elderly. *J R Soc Med*, **94**: 578–80. [PMID: 11691895]

Beulens JW, Kruidhof JS, Grobbee DE, Chaturvedi N, Fuller JH, Soedamah-Muthu SS (2008). Alcohol consumption and risk of microvascular complications in type 1 diabetes patients: the EURODIAB Prospective Complications Study. *Diabetologia*, **51**: 1631–8. [PMID: 18626626]

Cheyne EH, Sherwin RS, Lunt MJ, Cavan DA, Thomas PW, Kerr D (2004). Influence of alcohol on cognitive performance during mild hypoglycaemia; implications for Type 1 diabetes. *Diabet Med*, **21**: 230–7. [PMID: 15008832]

Cox DJ, Penberthy JK, Zrebiec J et al. (2003). Diabetes and driving mishaps: frequency and correlations from a multinational survey. *Diabetes Care*, **26**: 2329–34. [PMID: 12882857]

Cox DJ, Ford D, Gonder-Frederick L et al. (2009). Driving mishaps among individuals with type 1 diabetes: a prospective study. *Diabetes Care*, **32**: 2177–80. [PMID: 19940229]

DAFNE Study Group (2002). Training in flexible, intensive insulin management to enable dietary freedom in people with type 1 diabetes: dose adjustment for normal eating (DAFNE) randomised controlled trial. *BMJ*, **325**: 746. [PMID: 12364302]

Diabetes Control and Complications Trial Research Group (1995). Implementation of treatment protocols in the Diabetes Control and Complications Trial. *Diabetes Care*, **18**: 361–76. [PMID: 7555480]

Frier BM (2007). Living with hypoglycaemia. Chapter 14 in: *Hypoglycaemia in Clinical Diabetes*, 2nd edn. Frier BM, Fisher BM (eds). Wiley-Blackwell. ISBN: 978-0-42-001844-6

Graveling AJ, Warren RE, Frier BM (2004). Hypoglycaemia and driving in people with insulin-treated diabetes: adherence to recommendations for avoidance. *Diabet Med*, **21**: 1014–9. [PMID: 15317607]

Guelfi KJ, Jones TW, Fournier PA (2007). New insights into managing the risk of hypoglycaemia associated with intermittent high-intensity exercise in individuals with type 1 diabetes mellitus: implications for existing guidelines. *Sports Med*, **37**: 937–46. [PMID: 17953465]

Ismail D, Gebert R, Vuillermin PJ et al. (2006). Social consumption of alcohol in adolescents with Type 1 diabetes is associated with increased glucose lability, but not hypoglycaemia. *Diabet Med*, **23**: 830–3. [PMID: 16911618]

Juvenile Diabetes Research Foundation Continuous Glucose Monitoring Study Group. Tamborlane WV, Beck RW, Bode BW et al. (2008). Continuous glucose monitoring and intensive treatment of type 1 diabetes. *N Engl J Med*, **359**: 1464–76. [PMID: 18779236]

Juvenile Diabetes Research Foundation Continuous Glucose Monitoring Study Group. Tamborlane WV, Beck RW, Bode BW et al. (2010a). Effectiveness of continuous glucose monitoring in a clinical care environment: evidence from the Juvenile Diabetes Research Foundation continuous glucose monitoring (JDRF-CGM) trial. *Diabetes Care*, **33**: 17–22. [PMID: 19837791]

Juvenile Diabetes Research Foundation Continuous Glucose Monitoring Study Group. Tamborlane WV, Beck RW, Bode BW *et al.* (2010b). Prolonged nocturnal hypoglycemia is common during 12 months of continuous glucose monitoring in children and adults with type 1 diabetes. *Diabetes Care*, **33**: 1004–8. [PMID: 20200306]

Kahn R, Fonseca V (2008). Translating the A1C assay. *Diabetes Care*, **31**: 1704–7. [PMID: 18540045]

Kilpatrick ES, Rigby AS, Atkin SL (2008). HbA1c variability and the risk of microvascular complications in type 1 diabetes: data from the DCCT. *Diabetes Care*, **31**: 2198–202. [PMID: 18650371]

Lachin JM, Genuth S, Nathan DM, Zinman B, Rutledge BN; DCCT/EDIC Research Group (2008). Effect of glycemic exposure on the risk of microvascular complications in the Diabetes Control and Complications Trial—revisited. *Diabetes*, **57**: 995–1001. [PMID: 18223010]

Marliss EB, Vranic M (2002). Intense exercise has unique effects on both insulin release and its roles in glucoregulation: implications for diabetes. *Diabetes*, **51** (Suppl 1): S271–83. [PMID: 11815492]

Muller LM, Gorter KJ, Goudzwaard WL, Schellevis FG, Hoepelman AI, Rutten GE (2005). Increased risk of common infections in patients with type 1 and type 2 diabetes mellitus. *Clin Infect Dis*, **41**: 281–8. [PMID 16007521]

Nathan DM, Kuenen J, Borg R, Sheng H, Schoenfeld D, Heine RJ (2008) Translating the A1C assay into estimated average glucose values: A1C-Derived Average Glucose Study Group. *Diabetes Care*, **31**: 1473–8. [PMID: 18540046]

Rabasa-Lhoret R, Garon J, Langelier H, Poisson D, Chiasson JL (1999). Effects of meal carbohydrate content on insulin requirements in type 1 patients treated intensively with the basal-bolus (ultralente-regular) insulin regimen. *Diabetes Care*, **22**: 667–73. [PMID: 10332663]

Raccah D, Sulmont V, Reznik Y *et al.* (2009). Incremental value of continuous glucose monitoring when starting pump therapy in patients with poorly controlled type 1 diabetes: the RealTrend study. *Diabetes Care*, **32**: 2245–50. [PMID: 19767384]

Richardson T, Weiss M, Thomas P, Kerr D (2005). Day after the night before: influence of evening alcohol on risk of hypoglycemia in patients with type 1 diabetes. *Diabetes Care*, **28**: 1801–2. [PMID: 15983341]

Sämann A, Mühlhauser I, Bender R, Kloos Ch, Müller UA (2005). Glycaemic control and severe hypoglycaemia following training in flexible, intensive insulin therapy to enable dietary freedom in people with type 1 diabetes: a prospective implementation study. *Diabetologia*, **48**: 1965–70. [PMID 16132954]

Tamborlane W (2007). Triple jeopardy: nocturnal hypoglycemia after exercise in the young with diabetes. *J Clin Endocrinol Metab*, **92**: 815–6. [PMID: 17341578]

Vadén J, Forsblom C, Thorn LM et al. (2008). Physical activity and diabetes complications in patients with type 1 diabetes: the Finnish Diabetic Nephropathy (FinnDiane) Study. *Diabetes Care*, **31**: 230–2. [PMID:
17959867]

Wei C, Lunn DJ, Acerini CL et al. (2010). Measurement delay associated
with the Guardian RT continuous glucose monitoring system. *Diabet
Med*, **27**: 117–22. [PMID: 20121899]

Weinger K, Kinsley BT, Levy CJ et al. (1999). The perception of safe driving
ability during hypoglycemia in patients with type 1 diabetes mellitus.
Am J Med, **107**: 246–53. [PMID: 10492318]

Further reading

American Diabetes Association, Bantle JP, Wylie-Rosett J, Albright AL
et al. (2008). Nutrition recommendations and interventions for diabetes: a position statement of the American Diabetes Association. *Diabetes Care*, **31** (suppl 1): S61–78. [PMID: 18165339]

Franz MJ, Bantle JP, Beebe CA et al. (2003). Evidence-based nutrition
principles and recommendations for the treatment and prevention of
diabetes and related complications. *Diabetes Care*, **26** (Suppl 1): S51–
61. [PMID: 12502619]

Franz MJ, Boucher JL, Green-Pastors J, Powers MA (2008). Evidence-
based nutrition practice guidelines for diabetes and scope and stan-
dards of practice. *J Am Diet Assoc*, **108** (4 Suppl 1): S52–8. [PMID:
18358257]

Rachmiel M, Buccino J, Daneman D (2007). Exercise and Type 1 diabetes
mellitus in youth; review and recommendations. *Pediatr Endocrinol Rev*,
5: 656–65. [PMID: 18084160]

Sheard NF, Clark, NG, Brand-Miller JC et al. (2004). Dietary carbohydrate
(amount and type) in the prevention and management of diabetes: a
statement by the American Diabetes Association. *Diabetes Care*, **27**:
2266–71. [PMID: 15333500]

Sinclair AJ (ed) (2009). *Diabetes in old age,* 3rd edn. Wiley-Blackwell. [ISBN:
978-0-47-006562-4]

Smith SA, Poland GA; American Diabetes Association (2004). Influenza and
pneumococcal immunization in diabetes. *Diabetes Care*, **27** (Suppl 1):
S111–3. [PMID: 14693944]

Resources and websites

Textbooks

Bilous R, Donnelly R (eds) (2010). *Handbook of Diabetes*, 4th edn. Wiley-Blackwell. [ISBN: 978-1-40-518409-0]

DeFronzo RA, Ferrannini E, Keen H, Zimmet P (eds) (2004). *International Textbook of Diabetes*, 3rd edn. Wiley-Blackwell. [ISBN: 978-0-47-148655-8]

Donnelly R, Jonas J (eds) (2005) *Vascular Complications of Diabetes: Current Issues in Pathogenesis and Treatment,* 2nd edn. Wiley-Blackwell. [ISBN: 978-1-40-512785-1]

Frier BM, Fisher BM (eds) (2007). *Hypoglycaemia in Clinical Diabetes*, 2nd edn. Wiley-Blackwell. [ISBN: 978-0-47-001844-6]

Gill G (ed) (2004). *Unstable and Brittle Diabetes (Advances in Diabetes)*. Informa Healthcare. [ISBN: 978-1-84-184289-9]

Gill G, Pickup J, Williams G (eds) (2001). *Difficult Diabetes*. Wiley-Blackwell. [ISBN: 978-0-08-143129-3]

Holt RIG, Goldstein B, Flybjerg A, Cockram C (eds) (2010). *Textbook of Diabetes*, 4th edn. Wiley-Blackwell. [ISBN: 978-1-40-519181-4]

Inzucchi S, Porte D, Sherwin RS, Baron A (eds) (2005). *The Diabetes Mellitus Manual: A Primary Care Companion to Ellenberg and Rifkin's*, 6th edn. McGraw-Hill. [ISBN: 978-0-07-145129-3]

Kaufman FR (ed) (2008). *Medical Management of Type 1 Diabetes*, 5th revised edn. American Diabetes Association. [ISBN: 978-1-58-040309-2]

Krentz AJ (ed) (2004). *Emergencies in Diabetes: Diagnosis, Management and Prevention*. Wiley-Blackwell. [ISBN: 978-0-47-149814-8]

LeRoith D, Olefsky JM, Taylor SI (eds) (2003). *Diabetes Mellitus: A Fundamental and Clinical Text*, 3rd revised edn. Lippincott Williams & Wilkins. [ISBN: 978-0-78-174097-5]

Advanced self-help books

Bernstein RK (2007) *Dr Bernstein's Diabetes Solution: Complete Guide to Achieving Normal Blood Sugars*. Revised edn. Sphere. [ISBN: 978-0-31-616716-1]

Cheyette C, Balolia Y (2010). *Carbs and Cals: A Visual Guide to Carbohydrate Counting for People with Diabetes*, 3rd edn. Chello Publishing Limited. [ISBN: 978-0-95-644302-1]

Fox C, Kilvert A (2007). *Type 1 Diabetes: Answers at your Fingertips*, 6th revised edn. Class Publishing. [ISBN: 978-1-85-959175-8]

Hanas R (2006). Type 1 *Diabetes in Children, Adolescents and Young Adults* 3rd revised edn. Class Publishing. [ISBN: 978-1-85-959153-1]

Rubin AL (2008). *Type 1 Diabetes for Dummies.* Wiley-Blackwell. [ISBN 978-0-47-017811-9]

Scheiner G (2004). *Think Like a Pancreas: A Practical Guide to Managing Diabetes with Insulin.* Marlowe Diabetes Library: Marlowe & Co. [ISBN 978-1-56-924436-4]

Other books of related interest

Allgrove J, Swift P, Greene S (eds) (2007). *Evidence-Based Paediatric and Adolescent Diabetes.* Wiley-Blackwell. [ISBN: 978-1-40-515292-1]

Anderson BJ, Rubin RR (eds) (2002). *Practical Psychology for Diabetes Clinicians,* 2nd revised edn. American Diabetes Association. [ISBN: 978-1-58-040140-1]

Bennett MI (ed) (2006). *Neuropathic Pain (Oxford Pain Management Library).* Oxford University Press. [ISBN: 978-0-19-921418-2]

Bliss M (2007). *The Discovery of Insulin (Twenty-fifth Anniversary Edition).* Chicago University Press. [ISBN: 978-0-22-605899-3]

Dodson P (ed) (2009). *Diabetic Retinopathy (Oxford Diabetes Library).* Oxford University Press. [ISBN: 978-0-19-954496-7]

Feudtner C (2003). *Bittersweet: Diabetes, Insulin, and the Transformation of Illness (Studies in Social Medicine).* The University of North Carolina Press. [ISBN: 978-0-80-782791-8]

Fisher M. (ed) (2009). *Heart Disease and Diabetes (Oxford Diabetes Library).* Oxford University Press. [ISBN: 978-0-19-954372-4]

Greenhalgh T (2010). *How to Read a Paper: The Basics of Evidence-Based Medicine,* 4th edn. Wiley-Blackwell. [ISBN: 978-1-4443-3436-4]

Levy DM (2011) *Practical Diabetes Care,* 3rd edn. Wiley-Blackwell. [ISBN: 978-1-44-433385-5]

Pickup J (ed) (2009). *Insulin pump therapy and continuous glucose monitoring (Oxford Diabetes Library).* Oxford University Press. [ISBN: 978-0-19-956860-4]

Rodgers J (2008). *Using insulin pumps in diabetes: a guide for nurses and other health professionals.* Wiley-Blackwell. [ISBN: 978-0-47-005925-8]

Tesfaye S, Boulton A (eds) (2009). *Diabetic Neuropathy (Oxford Diabetes Library).* Oxford University Press. [ISBN: 978-0-19-955106-4]

National diabetes organizations

Diabetes UK: diabetes.org.uk

American Diabetes Association: diabetes.org

Diabetes Australia: diabetesaustralia.com.au

Diabetes New Zealand: diabetes.org.nz

Canadian Diabetes Association: diabetes.ca

National Institute for Health and Clinical Excellence (NICE) (nice.org.uk)

Technology appraisals relevant to Type 1 diabetes:

Continuous subcutaneous insulin infusion for the treatment of diabetes (review, 2008; TA151)

Diabetes (Types 1 and 2)—long-acting insulin analogues (2002; TA53)

Diabetes (Types 1 and 2)—patient education models (2003; TA60)

Clinical guidelines (2004)

Type 1 diabetes: diagnosis and management of Type 1 diabetes in adults

Type 1 diabetes: diagnosis and management of Type 1 diabetes in children and young adults

PG257. Allogeneic pancreatic islet-cell transplantation for Type 1 diabetes mellitus: guidance (2008)

Library resources

Medline: pubmed.gov

National Library of Health (UK): library.nhs.uk

Other websites

Children with Diabetes UK: childrenwithdiabetes.com.uk

DAFNE (Dose Adjustment for Normal Eating): dafne.uk.com

DCCT/EDIC: diabetes.niddk.nih.gov

Clinical trials in Type 1 diabetes prevention (close relatives and newly diagnosed): diabetestrialnet.org

Diabetes Research & Wellness Foundation: drwf.org.uk

DIRECT trials (2008; candesartan in diabetic retinopathy and microalbuminuria): direct-results.org

Insulin Dependent Diabetes Trust: iddtinternational.org

Juvenile Diabetes Research Foundation UK: JDRF.org.uk

Resources for exercise and athletes: runsweet.com

Index

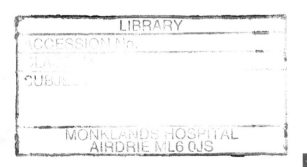